Challenging Operations

Tina:
for institutionalist
inspiration —
Thank you!
Kate

CHALLENGING

OPERATIONS

Medical Reform and Resistance in Surgery

Katherine C. Kellogg

UNIVERSITY OF CHICAGO PRESS

CHICAGO AND LONDON

Katherine Kellogg is associate professor of
organization studies at the MIT Sloan School
of Management.

The University of Chicago Press, Chicago 60637
The University of Chicago Press, Ltd., London
© 2011 by The University of Chicago
All rights reserved. Published 2011
Printed in the United States of America

20 19 18 17 16 15 14 13 12 11   1 2 3 4 5

ISBN-13: 978-0-226-43002-7 (cloth)
ISBN-13: 978-0-226-43003-4 (paper)
ISBN-10: 0-226-43002-2 (cloth)
ISBN-10: 0-226-43003-0 (paper)

Library of Congress Cataloging-in-Publication Data

Kellogg, Katherine C.
    Challenging operations: medical reform and
resistance in surgery / Katherine C. Kellogg
            p.   cm.
    Includes bibliographical references and index.
    ISBN-13: 978-0-226-43002-7 (cloth : alk paper)
    ISBN-10: 0-226-43002-2 (cloth : alk paper)
    ISBN-13: 978-0-226-43003-4 (pbk. : alk. paper)
    ISBN-10: 0-226-43003-0 (pbk. : alk. paper)
1. Hospitals—Medical staff. 2. Hours of labor.
I. Title.
    RA972.K455 2011
    362.11068'3—dc22

                                    2010052463

♾ The paper used in this publication meets the
minimum requirements of the American National
Standard for Information Sciences—Permanence
of Paper for Printed Library Materials,
ANSI Z39.48–1992.

For Randy, Chris, and Andrew

Contents

Preface

My interest in institutional change began when I read Lotte Bailyn's *Breaking the Mold* early in graduate school.[1] I remember being captivated by the idea that sometimes people conform to traditional ways of doing things not because it serves their interests, narrowly defined, but because these ways become so taken for granted that they are self-sustaining. Other times, people act according to widely accepted role expectations about how members of their class in good standing should behave. Over time, traditional ways become entrenched either because people can't conceive of alternatives or because they see them as inappropriate.

My knowledge of the institutional change literature was still developing when I attended a national conference on health care and, at lunch on the first day, sat next to Beth, the head of nursing at one of the hospitals I later studied. As we picked at the rubbery chicken and tough rolls one finds only at such events, she told me, "If you really want to study an interesting institutional change, you should study this upcoming change in resident work hours." "Surgery," she noted, "would be the place to study it." Surgical residents, who had historically worked 100–120 hours a week, would soon be required by new regulation to dramatically reduce their work hours to 80 in order to protect patient safety and residents' rights.

The issue sounded fascinating. In retrospect, it is not surprising I found it so. I had been working in the health care industry before graduate school and knew from experience how hard it is to accomplish change on the front lines inside health care organizations.

Beth offered to introduce me to the director of surgery at her hospital, and I took her up on it; through colleagues I was also able to make contact with surgery directors at two other hospitals in the same region. The three directors gave me permission to observe the implementation of the work-hours regulation as it occurred on the ground in their residency programs. By studying three hospitals responding to the same external pressure for change in long-standing practices, I hoped to learn how and why institutional change occurs.

When I first began to observe the residents inside these hospitals, I was amazed to find that some of them resisted the work-hours reduction (with no reduction in pay) that had been designed for their benefit. I couldn't get my head around two things: first, how eighty hours a week could be a *reduction* in work hours, and second, how anyone in their right mind could resist such a reduction. I was also struck by the exaggeratedly macho behavior of the residents who resisted change. I had friends in male-dominated professions, but the male swagger I observed in surgery was far beyond anything I had previously witnessed.

As I watched those I came to describe as Iron Men (they referred to long weekends spent on call as "Iron Man weekends"), I noted that they were the residents with the highest status in the surgical social world. Clearly their behavior was driven in part by a desire to protect this high status. But as I spent more time in the hospitals observing them, I came to understand (though not always agree with) the Iron Men for their strong commitment to their work. I learned that they resisted change not only to protect their status but also because they truly believed that the traditional ways of caring for patients and educating residents were the best ways.

As I went along, I discovered as well that not all residents accepted Iron Men dictates. Those I came to call reformers had greater interest in change than the Iron Men had, because their diverse social identities led them to be disadvantaged in the surgical social system. Unfortunately for these would-be reformers, their early attempts to individually modify work practices in everyday encounters failed because the defenders refused to go along.

My search to better understand how power figured into institutional change in surgery led me to the work of neo-institutionalists, law and society theorists, social movement theorists, and medical sociologists. This research pointed to the key actors, processes, and resources that push defenders of the status quo inside organizations to change work practices. It helped me make sense of how changes in the hospitals' environment helped bring about change in daily work practices by both pressuring internal defenders and assisting internal reformers.

But the processes of change I observed at the three hospitals did not fit well with the processes described by any of these theories. In attempting to change long-standing practices, reformers at the three hospitals did more than question surgical institutions in the abstract; instead, they struck at the very heart of each defender by challenging the traditional work practices defenders were skilled in and the deeply held beliefs defenders used to justify their position atop the existing social hierarchy. Defenders had a vested interest in maintaining the status quo, and they protected their traditional practices by aggressively retaliating in the face of change efforts. Change or stasis at the three hospitals was the result of fierce contestation on the ground between defenders of the traditional practices and insurgent reformers.

I found that to explain the different change trajectories and outcomes at the three hospitals, I needed to understand the collective combat processes used by defenders of the status quo and reformers in their day-to-day workplace encounters. And I needed to understand the micro-level resources available to defenders and reformers within each hospital. As I tell the tale that follows, I seek to explain what led to the different outcomes at the three hospitals and, in so doing, advance a *micro-institutional approach* to the study of institutional change.

Introduction

On the night of March 4, 1984, Alva and Sidney Zion, a prominent Manhattan couple, brought their 18-year-old daughter, Libby, to the emergency room at New York Hospital–Cornell Medical Center. She had a high fever and was delirious. She shook and moved her arms and legs erratically. Sidney Zion called his own doctor . . . and asked him to come to the hospital. . . . Instead, he referred Libby's care to the doctors in training on duty that night.

. . . Libby's fever went down, her agitation lessened, and she was calm. A medical resident told her parents to go home, that she would be all right. Soon after that Libby's fever rose again, and she thrashed about her bed and pulled out her IV needle. A nurse . . . called the intern to come right away. The intern, overwhelmed with too many patients, probably exhausted after a straight 36 hours of work, delayed coming. Libby died at 7:30 the next morning. (*Washington Post*, 1995)[1]

Libby Zion's death received national attention, in part due to the efforts of her father, Sidney Zion. Sidney Zion was an author, a columnist at the *Daily News*, a former reporter for the *New York Times* and the *New York Post*, and a former federal prosecutor.[2] In response to Libby's death, he and other patient safety and resident rights reformers began what would become a decades-long fight to regulate resident work hours.

The reformers pressed for and won an unusual New York grand jury investigation of the case. The grand jury directly blamed neither the hospital nor the physicians for the medication error that led to Zion's death, but it did find fault with the system of medical training that allowed her death to occur. Residents were routinely working more than 100 hours per week and providing patient care continuously for 30- to 40-hour periods. The grand jury cited exhausted, sleep-deprived residents and the lack of supervision as serious potential dangers to patients. They found New York State's method of training doctors, one that was in common use across the country, to be counterproductive to providing quality medical care.[3]

Shortly after the grand jury's report was released, the prestigious *New England Journal of Medicine* focused its spotlight on the resident work hours controversy. Commenting on the report in a special issue of the journal, one doctor wrote that "house officers (residents) are overworked, sleep-deprived and unduly stressed. The result is damage to their well being, to medical education, to patient care, and to the entire profession. . . . Few would choose to ride in a car driven by a resident coming off a 36-hour shift. It should come as no surprise that the public would question the ability of sleep-deprived residents to make life-and-death decisions."[4]

In March 1987, the New York State commissioner of health appointed nine distinguished New York physicians to an advisory committee to analyze the grand jury findings. The blue-ribbon committee, chaired by Bertrand Bell of Brooklyn's Einstein Medical Center, reviewed the report and issued recommendations for graduate medical education reform, one of which was that residents' workweeks should be limited to eighty hours. In 1989, its recommendations, commonly known as the Bell Regulations, became part of the New York State health code.[5]

Since the Bell Regulations limited hours for residents only in New York State, patient rights and resident rights reformers began to press for national regulations. Reformers raised public awareness of these issues by drawing attention to the voluminous scientific literature on the cognitive and functional deficits associated with sleep deprivation; this literature shows that sleep deprivation negatively affects attention, memory, problem solving, and decision making.[6] One study reported that interns made almost twice as many errors reading electrocardiograms after an extended (24-hour or more) work shift as after a night of sleep.[7] Another study showed that surgical residents made up to twice the number of technical errors in the performance of simulated laparoscopic surgical procedures after working overnight as after a night of sleep.[8] Reformers noted that the literature as a whole demonstrated that sleep deprivation causes substantial decrements in physicians' performance of discrete neurocognitive and simulated clinical tasks.[9]

In addition to drawing on the scientific literature, reformers used medical providers' own accounts to raise public concerns about the effects of sleep deprivation on patient care. An article in the *Los Angeles Times* quoted a surgeon as saying, "It's not unusual to see residents fall asleep in the operating room, sometimes while holding scalpels or other instruments." One resident confessed, "You actually start wishing patients would die so you could get some sleep."[10]

Reformers argued that patients were not the only ones at risk. They pointed to scientific studies showing that residents suffered increased motor vehicle accidents when fatigued and increased exposure to blood-borne pathogens from needle punctures at night.[11] Residents also were more vulnerable to depression than the general population and were more likely to suffer complications during pregnancy, including giving birth to premature or underweight infants.[12] Reformers quoted residents who disclosed that they frequently nodded off while driving home. "I don't think that you would find a resident anyplace who has not had that experience," Mark Levy, executive director of the Committee of Interns and Residents, told the *New York Post*. "Some will describe falling asleep on the highway." Valentin Barbuescu, a resident at Jacobi Hospital in the Bronx, was killed when his car ran off the road and hit a tree in rural Pennsylvania.[13]

In addition to raising public awareness of the hazards of long resident work hours, reformers launched a national campaign to establish enforceable work-hour limits. In 2001, a coalition of reformer organizations—Public Citizen, the American Medical Student Association, and the Committee of Interns and Residents—wrote a petition to the Occupational Safety and Health Administration (OSHA) asking for such limits.[14] Reformer organizations collaborated with Congressman John Conyers of Michigan and Senator Jon Corzine of New Jersey to introduce the Patient and Physician Safety and Protection Act in the US House and Senate. The bill would have authorized the US secretary of Health and Human Services to set regulations on resident duty hours and supervision and provide for whistleblower protection. It also would have levied fines for nonadherence and provided funding to help training facilities meet regulations.[15]

Not surprisingly, many in the medical community were unmoved by these calls for reform. Indeed, surgeons created a countermovement, and the institutional home they used to mount their resistance was the highly respected American College of Surgeons. At their annual meetings, surgeons articulated their opposition to the proposed work hour limits and built solidarity networks for collective resistance.

In conference presentations, journal articles, position papers, and media reports, defenders of the status quo painted their critics as outsiders who did not understand the needs of patients and residents. If hours were reduced, they said, there would have to be more handoffs of work between residents. They drew attention to the scientific literature that shows that handoffs are worse for patient care than tired surgeons, because handoffs disrupt continuity of care. One study showed that the 1989 New York State work-hour restrictions were associated with delayed ordering of tests and more frequent in-hospital complications.[16] Another study found that coverage by a physician from another resident team was strongly associated with adverse events that continuity would presumably have prevented.[17]

Learning the valuable skills of a surgeon, defenders argued, required spending as many hours in the hospital as possible during residency. If residents worked fewer hours, they would not learn that they must provide care for their patients whenever it was needed, regardless of time of day or inconvenience to themselves; residents would develop a shift-worker mentality rather than an ethic of commitment to the patient.[18] Moreover, reducing resident work hours would require the elimination of some rotations, narrowing residents' scope of knowledge; it would also require the elimination of operating days, significantly diminishing surgical case experience. Lazar Greenfield, chair of the Residency Review Committee for Surgery, said: "The potential [with an eighty-hour workweek] is to lose every third day of operative experience — the cases the residents are looking forward to performing after being on call the night before."[19]

The use of conflicting scientific data by the reform movement and the countermovement naturally raises the question of whose claims about patient safety were more accurate. On the one hand, little research either then or now has focused specifically on physician fatigue and its relationship to patient safety. New resident schedules designed to reduce sleep deprivation may simultaneously introduce discontinuities in care. On the other hand, despite the lack of data collected in clinical settings, there is a large number of scientific studies on the cognitive and functional deficits induced by fatigue. In addition, a landmark study in the 2004 *New England Journal of Medicine* found that reducing medical residents' work hours during rotations in the intensive care unit resulted in a significant reduction in medical errors.[20] As I discuss in my concluding chapter, the evidence that does exist concerning resident safety and the risk of errors when fatigued led the Institute of Medicine in 2008 to argue for "strong and prompt action" to improve patient safety.[21]

In this book I do not try to adjudicate between the claims of the movement and those of the countermovement about the effects of long work hours versus handoffs on patient care. Qualitative research methods are not well suited to answering such questions. And while such measurements are valuable and necessary, they don't tell the whole story. The ethnographic study presented in this book is extremely well suited to answering a different set of important questions—how and why reforms like resident work-hours reform are actually implemented (or not) inside organizations.

THE BEGINNINGS

To begin answering these questions, we need a bit of history about the origins of the work-hours reform. The countermovement successfully preempted national legislation that would have made it illegal for hospitals to require long resident work hours by arguing that only the American Council for Graduate Medical Education (ACGME), the organization responsible for oversight of residency training, should be responsible for work-hours restrictions. OSHA agreed and rejected the reformers' petition. Before Congress had a chance to consider the Patient and Physician Safety Bill, the ACGME announced a new set of rules for all medical and surgical specialties.

The ACGME required work hours for all residents to be limited to eighty per week, averaged over a four-week period, starting in July 2003. In addition, residents were to be provided one day in seven free from all educational and clinical responsibilities. This, too, was to be averaged over a four-week period, including call activities. A ten-hour period was required between all daily duty periods and after in-house call.[22]

In theory, the ACGME regulation had real bite. ACGME accreditation was required for a residency program to get reimbursement for training residents from the Centers for Medicare and Medicaid Services. These reimbursements totaled $8 billion annually.[23] Perhaps even more significant, individuals who graduated from residency programs could sit for board certification only if their residency programs were accredited. ACGME had signaled its potential power by threatening to take away accreditation from the Yale medical school when inspectors found that its residents were not complying with previous ACGME guidelines regarding resident training.[24]

However, from the start reformers were skeptical of the new ACGME regulations. Bertrand Bell wrote: "It would not be gratuitous to suggest that the ACGME was really not particularly worried about reducing error by sleep deprived residents but rather they are very interested in forestalling government interference with graduate medical education."[25] A June 2002 editorial in the *New York Times* noted that "despite the tough talk, the council faces an inherent conflict of interest. Its board is dominated by the trade associations for hospitals, doctors and medical schools, all of which benefit from the cheap labor provided by medical residents. For violations there is little reason to expect that the ACGME will be little more than an apologist for the industry."[26]

Hospital administrators across the country, unsure whether the ACGME would treat noncompliance lightly, began to develop formal programs that would allow them to comply with the new rules. Because they could not receive federal reimbursement for hiring new residents to staff these new programs, many hospitals cut the number of resident rotations to free up existing residents to work on "night float teams," coming in each night so that day residents could leave instead of having to stay on call every third night.[27] In July 2004, twelve months after the new regulation went into effect, ACGME regulators reviewing hospital reports found that 95 percent of hospitals reviewed were in full compliance with the new regulations.[28]

But reporters who managed to talk to residents and investigate specific residency programs found that "full compliance" was a sham. Soon after the regulation took effect, residents across the country began sending anonymous e-mails to the press expressing their frustration. At many hospitals, residents were told fairly explicitly to falsify the timesheets that the ACGME used to measure compliance.[29] One resident at Chicago's Northwestern Memorial Hospital vented anonymously to *The New Physician*, a medical journal: "I continue to work 35 to 45 hour shifts and I was instructed not to go home post-call. At the current rate, I will also definitely average over 80 hours per week. . . . When the residents asked our Chairman about this issue, we were asked to 'lie' in our reporting of work hours. Fearing retribution from the faculty, I'm sure the residents will comply on paper but not in actuality."[30] A study in *JAMA*, which used anonymous surveys of first-year residents to measure compliance with the regulation the year it took effect, reported that interns in 67 percent of hospital general surgery departments said they were working more than eighty hours per week.[31] Since residents may have been nervous about accurately reporting their work hours for fear of retribution, surveys such as this one, even when completely anonymous, likely overestimated compliance.

Most hospitals, the data show, did not change their traditional practices. But some did, and the central concern of this book is to explain the reasons for such different outcomes.

SIMILAR HOSPITALS, DIFFERENT OUTCOMES

The process that ultimately led to new regulation followed a familiar script: An adverse event provides reformers fighting for the rights of a disadvantaged group with a new political opportunity. They use the event to reframe long-standing work practices as problematic, mobilize reformer networks and organizations, and garner resources for change. They fight to protect organizations' customers or employees and, when successful, best opponents and win new regulation. In response to the pressure for change, organizations adopt formal programs to implement change in concert with reformer goals. The public's expectations run high.

For those who support reform, however, the story's ending is often less than satisfying. While reformers have won new or modified regulations, these regulations do not automatically force organizations to alter practices. When regulations run counter to the interests of powerful organization members, organizations may create believable displays of conformity but decouple these programs from actual daily practices.[32] Thus, in response to external pressure for change, some organizations make real change but others engage in merely symbolic compliance or make no change at all.

Why do some organizations change and others not? *Challenging Operations* builds on decades of social science work on institutional change to answer this question. Most prior research provides valuable insights into how institutional change happens at the macro level of professions, industries, and countries. But the key finding of this book is that even the most dramatic change at the macro level comes to nothing if it is not collectively embraced in practice by those who must do their work in a new way. By looking at the macro level, we can understand how and why institutional change is *initiated*—but until we look at the micro level, we cannot explain how and why institutional change is ultimately *accomplished*.

I was able to gain ethnographic access to study what happened in response to the new work-hours regulation in the surgery departments of three hospitals—Advent, Bayshore, and Calhoun (pseudonyms). Each of the hospitals issued me its version of surgical scrubs, and over the course of two and a half years, from January 2002 through July 2004, I studied how the residents and staff surgeons on the general surgery services did their work.

I soon discovered that changing the daily work practices targeted by the regulation proved difficult because it required challenging long-standing beliefs, roles, and authority relations. While change processes at the three hospitals were similar for the first several months, over the course of the study, members acted quite differently in each hospital and outcomes diverged radically. First, Advent and Calhoun reformers successfully built coalitions across different work positions to collectively challenge defenders of the status quo, while Bayshore reformers did not. Then, after an initially successful mobilization at both Advent and Calhoun, Advent reformers effectively maintained their coalition in the face of defender attempts to divide it, while at Calhoun reformers did not. Why?

MACRO-LEVEL EXPLANATIONS

My search to understand the different institutional change outcomes at the three hospitals led me to four different theories: neo-institutional theory, law and society theory, social movement theory, and medical sociology. As I will discuss below, each of these theories highlights different aspects of institutional change, but they are similar in their explanation of change as stemming predominantly from macro-level actors, macro-level processes, and macro-level resources. (Readers less interested in theoretical arguments may want to skip ahead to the section titled "A Micro-institutional Approach.")

NEO-INSTITUTIONAL THEORY

Neo-institutional theory offers some explanations for why institutional change outcomes in the three hospitals may have differed. In their reviews of the neo-institutionalist literature, Paul DiMaggio, Neil Fligstein, Royston Greenwood, Christine Oliver, Walter Powell, Kerstin Sahlin, Roy Suddaby, Richard Scott, Pamela Tolbert, and Lynn Zucker explain that change in long-standing practices is difficult because institutions constrain behavior by threatening punishment for noncompliance, defining what is good, right, and appropriate, and providing shared logics of action that make new behaviors inconceivable.[33] Given these constraints, institutions are relatively resistant to change. Still, change can occur when macro-level actors alter long-standing practices for their own benefit.[34] The actors who can most readily initiate changes are those on the periphery of an industry; they are "institutional entrepreneurs." Because they are not deeply embedded in the industry, they are less constrained by the industry's ways of doing and thinking than are more central actors.[35] Central actors are important, of course, but this is because they are the ones who ultimately help innovations become accepted after they are introduced by the institutional entrepreneurs.[36]

Institutional entrepreneurs accomplish institutional change through the macro-level processes of theorizing new practices, legitimating them, and disseminating them throughout the field.[37] They theorize new practices such as using museums for education (in addition to conservation and collection) or using accounting firms for business advisory services (in addition to audit and accounting services).[38] They legitimate such new practices by using their social skill to link them to logics valued by practitioners.[39] And they disseminate the practices across organizations by enacting new regulation, circulating new norms through professional networks, and developing new ideologies.[40] Some organizations are more likely to embrace practices introduced by institutional entrepreneurs than others, and often this is determined by the degree of their exposure to macro-level pressures and resources. Different organizational environments have different levels of functional pressures (perceived problems associated with current practices), political pressures (shifts in interests or underlying power distributions), and social pressures (differentiation of groups), and thus some accept new practices much more rapidly than others.[41] Organizational characteristics like size, visibility, and identity can also make it harder or easier for new practices to be identified or to take hold.[42] And top managers' interests, experience, or identities may make a crucial difference.[43]

Neo-institutional theorists would likely explain the different outcomes I observed by suggesting that the three hospitals must have been targeted by different kinds of institutional entrepreneurs or affected by different theorization and legitimation processes, or that their environmental, organizational, or top manager characteristics must have been different. However, as I will explain in more detail in the following chapters, the hospitals I studied were similar on all of these dimensions.

LAW AND SOCIETY THEORY

A second theory that sheds light on the difference in outcomes among the three hospitals is law and society theory. In their overviews of the interactions between law and organizations, Frank Dobbin, Lauren Edelman, Carol Heimer, Alexandra Kalev, Erin Kelly, Calvin Morrill, Susan Silbey, Robin Stryker, and Mark Suchman note that law is not an external, authoritative, and unambiguous force acting on organizations; rather, law is shaped through the interactions of professionals, legislators, and the judiciary.[44] Often new laws have broad mandates and do not specify clear standards of compliance.[45] In the face of such ambiguity, macro-level actors such as professional groups of personnel officers or lawyers act for change both because they are committed to change-oriented ideals and in order to increase their power vis-à-vis other groups of professionals.[46]

Professionals create change in organizational practices through macro-level processes such as interpreting new laws and setting up new compliance programs for organizations. For example, professionals responded to civil rights laws by inventing internal labor markets, grievance procedures, and sex discrimination and maternity leave policies.[47] They used venues such as journals, conferences, and networks to hone these programs.[48] To persuade employers to adopt them, professionals often cast them in terms of efficiency rather than employee rights.[49]

According to law and society theorists, organizational response to new laws is shaped by differences in environmental, organizational, and top and mid-level manager characteristics. Organizations are more likely to adopt programs to comply with regulation when legal objectives are clear, sanctions for noncompliance are strong, and beliefs and norms support compliance as the right and proper thing to do.[50] Large, highly visible organizations, particularly nonprofit or public agencies, are more receptive to new programs, as are organizations that have separate personnel offices.[51] Finally, organizations are more likely to adopt new compliance programs when institutional pressures coincide with the interests of top- and mid-level managers.[52]

But in the case of resident work-hours regulation, differences in the involvement of professional groups, the formulation of new compliance programs, environmental, organizational, or top and mid-level manager characteristics cannot account for why Advent was able to reform its everyday practices but Bayshore and Calhoun were not. For, as I will show, the hospitals were similar in all these aspects.

SOCIAL MOVEMENT THEORY

Social movement theorists also inform our understanding of why different organizations succeed or fail at reforming themselves. In their discussions of the interactions between social movements and organizations, Elisabeth Clemens, Gerald Davis, Heather Haveman, Michael Lounsbury, Doug McAdam, Calvin Morrill, Hayagreeva Rao, Richard Scott, Sarah Soule, and Mayer Zald have demonstrated how social movements are important engines of institutional change.[53] In the social movement view, institutional change occurs because reformers seek to challenge the advantaged position of powerful defenders, around whose interests the field revolves.[54]

Reformers facilitate change through macro-level processes of framing, mobilizing, and creating political opportunity.[55] They develop frames such as "equal pay for equal work" and identities such as "working mothers" that diagnose problems, specify collective actions to solve those problems, and provide reformers inside organizations with appropriate behaviors vis-à-vis other actors.[56] They build mobilizing structures like social movement organizations and networks that afford reformers the community and solidarity necessary to take the risks associated with protest.[57] And they create political opportunities like new regulations or boycotts that give reformers leverage to make new claims.[58]

Organizations respond differentially to social movements depending on differences in the strength of the macro-level resources provided to reformers inside organizations.[59] Strong frames and identities are those that resonate with the beliefs of those within the organization.[60] Strong mobilizing structures are accessible to internal reformers yet often in locations separate from their workplace.[61] And strong political opportunities are those that help lower the risks of collective action inside organizations or increase the likelihood of its success.[62] Organizations also respond differently to social movements depending on how committed their top managers are to reform. When managers are opposed to social movement goals, they can deny promotions, set up counterorganizations, and provide official interpretive responses to challenges that result in raising the costs of reform attempts inside their organizations.[63] On the other hand, when they support social movement reform, they can develop new policies consistent with reform and commit important resources to facilitate its implementation.[64]

But differences among social movement actors, framing and mobilizing processes, and resources available to reformers inside organizations cannot account for the different outcomes at the three hospitals. As I will explain in more detail in the following chapters, these were the same across hospitals.

MEDICAL SOCIOLOGY

Finally, medical sociology offers an important perspective that could help explain the different success in implementing medical reform at the three hospitals. In their overviews of control over medical practice, Andrew Abbott, Chloe Bird, Phillip Brown, Peter Conrad, Eliot Freidson, Allen Fremont, Donald Light, Frederic Hafferty, Jill Quadagno, and Paul Starr have provided pictures of the macro-level actors, processes, and resources involved in challenges to the US medical profession's dominance over time.[65] Social movements, the government, corporate buyers, corporate sellers, nonphysician healthcare providers, and consumers—have frequently tried to make inroads into physicians' monopoly on medical practice.[66] But powerful physician associations like the American Medical Association (AMA) have historically met challenges to physicians' professional boundaries with strong resistance.[67]

For much of the twentieth century, physicians were able to maintain control of their expert knowledge and the high-status position this knowledge afforded using credentialing, registration, and licensing.[68] They fought particularly hard to protect control of training programs because these programs not only taught required technical skills but also formalized the knowledge and skills claimed by the profession and therefore underwrote the intellectual basis for its jurisdictional claims.[69] In addition, medical training provided new recruits with a moral education crucial to their assimilation of professional attitudes, a professional conscience, and professional standards of practice.[70] Yet escalating costs and wide variation in patient care practices in the United States in the 1950s and 1960s led to a decline in public trust in medical professionals and an increase in activism for change.[71] In the face of such pressures, one of the ways physician associations tried to regain the public's trust while protecting their professional dominance was by adopting new standards.[72]

Yet new regulations and standards in medicine often result in only minor changes in actual clinical behavior.[73] As Renee Anspach, Marc Berg, Charles Bosk, Daniel Chambliss, Carol Heimer, Lisa Staffen, Stephan Timmermans, and Robert Zussman have shown, even in situations where the courts and legislatures have mandated the protection of patients' rights, physicians have maintained their autonomy in practice by keeping patients and families on the periphery of decision making.[74] Differences in macro-level resources have been shown to lead to differences in the implementation of regulations and standards; change in response to regulation varies because of differences in the content of regulation (different regulations afford different costs and benefits to frontline clinicians) and differences in groups involved (different groups benefit differently from each regulation).[75]

One way to explain the different outcomes I observed at the three hospitals, then, would be to suggest that the hospitals were exposed to different social movements or interest groups, different kinds of jurisdictional challenges, or different types of regulation. Yet as I will detail, the three hospitals were evenly matched on these dimensions.

A MICRO-INSTITUTIONAL APPROACH

While these four theories help us understand institutional change, they cannot explain why the change outcomes of Advent, Bayshore, and Calhoun differed. If differences in macro-level actors, processes, and resources cannot explain the differences in outcomes at the three hospitals, what can? The *micro-institutional approach* developed in this book provides a different and, in this case, more revealing perspective on institutional change than does the predominant macro-institutional approach. To support my claim that institutional change occurs not only at the macro level but also at the micro level, I make three key arguments.

First, I demonstrate that for institutional change to occur, in addition to external reformers such as institutional entrepreneurs, professionals, social movements, and interest groups, coalitions of reformers inside organizations must fight for it. And for these internal reformers to succeed, they need to build and maintain coalitions across different work positions and social identities, along with using resources provided by external reformers.

Second, I show that differences in institutional change outcomes are driven by differences in micro-level processes as much as by differences in macro-level ones. While theorizing and disseminating, developing new compliance models, framing and mobilizing, and fighting jurisdictional battles are clearly important for change, they must be accompanied by face-to-face collective combat on the ground inside organizations for change to occur.

Third, I argue that institutional change outcomes are shaped not only by differences in macro-level resources originating outside the organization but also by micropolitical resources available to reformers and defenders inside specific organizations. While environmental, organizational, and top-manager characteristics are important, organization members' capacity to resist or press for change is shaped by particular resources available in the local context.

IMPLICATIONS FOR MEDICAL REFORM

My aims in this book are several. Certainly the book has important implications for theorists, but I will also make recommendations for external reformers, medical administrators, and providers interested in implementing medical reform. Over the last several decades, concerns about rapidly rising medical costs, uneven access to medical care, sick care rather than preventive care, little public accountability, and a dearth of primary care physicians have led political leaders to engage in battles over healthcare reform. In 2010, these battles led to the passing of historic healthcare legislation.

But this is by no means the first time reformers have tried to affect medical care. Numerous other attempts to improve healthcare quality and control medical costs—through health maintenance organizations (HMOs), peer review organizations, diagnostic related groups (DRGs), and evidence-based medicine—have fallen far short of expectations.[76] This book points to some of the difficulties of reforming health care on the ground and offers some concrete recommendations for how it can be done effectively.

AN OVERVIEW OF THE METHODOLOGY

To develop these claims, I draw on ethnographic data from my two-and-a-half-year field study of surgery departments. My methodological strategy is comparative ethnography.

Data were collected using a combination of ethnographic observation of and interviews with residents, attendings, and directors in surgery at the three hospitals.[77] At Advent and Bayshore, I spent fifteen months following residents in surgery as they did their daily work. Among other activities, I followed residents as they visited patients twice daily on rounds, I scrubbed in on surgeries, and I slept overnight in family waiting rooms next to the resident call rooms so that I could get up with residents in the middle of the night. I regularly ate breakfast, lunch, and dinner with residents, fraternized with them in the residents' lounges, and attended resident parties and weekly drinking evenings to understand the surgical social world and immerse myself in its customs and habits.

I noted early on that the residents I was studying seemed to be choosing sides in a fight. Since I wanted to get both sides of the story, I tried to be careful not to affiliate predominantly with either reformers or defenders, and I spent a lot of time fretting about whether I was doing this successfully. I had received the good advice that I should position myself low in the surgical hierarchy to start, because while moving up the chain would be easy, moving down would be difficult: those lower down would worry that I would betray their confidences to their superiors.[78] Therefore I dressed as an intern (first-year resident) and began my observations by following interns. This positioning turned out to be helpful, because interns did not initially choose sides in the fight; instead, they did their work and kept their mouths shut, and I did the same.

While I tried not to align with either reformers or defenders, I did feel the need to make it clear that I was on the side of the residents rather than the directors. Once I began my observations, I did my best to avoid the director at each hospital who had granted me research access. Directors saw residents as a group in weekly Mortality and Morbidity conferences and in special teaching sessions. In these meetings I purposely did not talk to the directors. In fact, at one of the hospitals a director did not recognize me, dressed as I was as an intern, and called on me in a teaching session to answer one of his surgical questions. I sheepishly reminded him that I was just a researcher. Everyone laughed as he sharply told me that this was no excuse.

My early field notes show that I spent a lot of time worrying that I had offended this person or that person, trying to make sense of the fact that someone who had recently been very nice was now inexplicably acting chilly, and so on. But general surgical services are extremely busy, and residents are used to being followed around by medical students. I felt my presence affected the phenomena I was observing in only insignificant ways, and my informants were usually quite willing to share their thoughts and feelings. Over time they got more and more comfortable with me, and my reception went from "Oh no, the researcher is following me today" to "Hey Kate, let's grab lunch."

To establish a baseline regarding the way work was done before any changes were made, I observed residents three months before new compliance programs were introduced at Advent and Bayshore. For the first eight months, I spent an average of twenty hours a week on site at each hospital.

After eight months of observation at Bayshore, because the work practice targeted for change remained unchanged and stable, for the final seven months of fieldwork I scaled back my time spent there to approximately five hours per week. At Advent, where the targeted work practice had still not stabilized, I continued to spend twenty hours or more per week on site.

My work at Calhoun was based primarily on interviews and started a year later than that at Advent and Bayshore. In chapter 2, I explain why the timing difference in my research at the three hospitals cannot explain the difference in outcomes. My familiarity with surgical culture and work practices, gleaned from the time at Advent and Bayshore, enabled me to fit in quickly at Calhoun. Further, I observed a good deal of everyday life at Calhoun by spending time with groups of two and three residents outside of interviews in the surgical resident lounge and hospital cafeteria. My interviews were designed as extended ethnographic interviews, asking questions primarily about work practices and significant (to the interviewee) events.[79] I conducted ninety-three semistructured interviews with residents, attendings, and directors at two different points: once before their new compliance program was introduced and again twelve months later, at the end of the residency year.[80]

My analysis of data collected at the three hospitals consisted of both informal analysis during my fieldwork and more formal analysis once data collection was complete.[81] While I was in the field, I wrote weekly memos creating preliminary categories and groupings to explain what I was finding. On occasion I also left the field for several weeks to review what I was learning and construct interpretations to discover where I needed to concentrate future observations. Once I finished my data collection, I entered all of my field notes and interview transcripts into ATLAS/ti, a qualitative data analysis program, and began to develop the description and theoretical accounts that appear in this book.

OUTLINE OF THE BOOK

The book is divided into two parts. Part I looks at the pre-change world of surgery, and part II examines the change attempts themselves. In chapter 1, I describe what life was like before the change for surgical residents working 100–120 hours a week. Chapter 2 provides data on the organizational characteristics of the three hospitals and the plans they made to comply with the regulation. Chapter 3 explains why attending surgeons and even some residents in the three hospitals resisted a change designed, as noted, to improve both safety for the patients and the quality of education and work life for the residents. Chapter 4 characterizes the internal reformers and explains why they questioned traditional surgical practices.

Having outlined the similarities in surgical residency at the three hospitals, I then turn in part II to the collective combat processes that defenders and reformers inside the hospitals used to try to maintain or change traditional practices in response to the regulation. Chapter 5 details how defenders initially resisted change at all three hospitals. Chapter 6 shows how relational spaces at Advent and Calhoun allowed reformers in these two hospitals to build a cross-position coalition to collectively challenge defenders, while at Bayshore reformers did not. Chapter 7 examines how the threat posed by a reformer subgroup played an important role in the failure of change at Calhoun. And chapter 8 describes the process that reformers used to force defenders to accept practice change at Advent. In the conclusion, I summarize the micro-level processes used by defenders and reformers at the three hospitals and discuss the book's more general implications for our theoretical understanding of institutional change and our practical understanding of medical reform implementation.

PART ONE

- -

THE WORLD AT 120 HOURS A WEEK

1

A Day in the Life
of an Intern

When Anne (a pseudonym)[1] crept out the back door of her apartment building, a blast of cold, damp air hit her face. It was dark, 3:50 a.m. She closed
the door quietly behind her and, shivering in her threadbare lab coat and
scrub pants, found her way to her beat-up gray Honda. Anne pulled out
of the parking lot and drove slowly down Springdale Avenue. At the traffic light, she yielded to the urge to let her head fall back on the headrest.
Abruptly, she forced herself awake, leveling her head, straightening her
arms against the steering wheel, and opening her mouth in a large yawn. It
was only a five-minute drive from her apartment to the hospital, but she had
fallen asleep waiting at traffic lights more times than she could remember.
She was luckier than one of her fellow surgical residents: he had been in a
car accident after drifting across a highway median line while driving to see
his girlfriend on a rare weekend off.

In the United States, doctors like Anne who graduate from medical
school receive the degree of medical doctor (MD) but are not permitted to
practice medicine on their own. Those who hope to become surgeons must
complete a five-year clinical training program (often with an additional two
years in the laboratory) called surgical residency. During this time, under
the tutelage of surgical "attendings" (staff surgeons), residents learn to diag-

nose patients, recommend potential surgeries, operate on patients, and provide post-surgical care. After the completion of their residency programs, they can enter into surgical practice.

Anne pulled into the low-ceilinged hospital garage and parked. She absent-mindedly buttoned up her white lab coat and pulled back her wiry red hair into a black scrunchie as she walked up the sidewalk to the hospital entrance.

I met Anne as she walked through the hospital's [2] revolving doors at 4:00 a.m. Like her, I was dressed in surgical scrubs, a lab coat, and leather medical clogs. And I was bleary-eyed and tired like her, too. I marveled, as I had many times before, at Anne and the other residents' ability to arrive at work on time every morning while keeping up the punishing schedule of every third night on call.

To effectively study institutional change as it occurred on the ground, I needed to begin by establishing a baseline of how work had traditionally been done. That is why I was there on that damp June morning before any new compliance program had been introduced, observing Anne, an intern (first-year resident) assigned to the surgical oncology service that month.

A janitor pushed a mop across the gleaming marble floor of the dark, empty lobby and a stern-looking woman at the security desk glanced at our badges as Anne and I made our way toward the elevator bank. We took the elevator up to the eighth floor and I followed Anne to one of the call rooms. She entered a five-digit code on the metal keypad, and we went in. Light from the hallway fell across the body of a resident, asleep under a white cotton blanket. It was Ryan, the senior resident who was working on the oncology service with Anne.

At Anne's hospital, as in surgical residency programs at other hospitals across the country, teams of "chiefs" (fifth-year residents), "seniors" (second-, third-, and fourth-year residents), and "interns" (first-year residents) took care of ten to twenty patients on each general surgery service (e.g., surgical oncology, vascular, gastrointestinal [GI]). A team was typically composed of a chief, a senior, and an intern. Chiefs formulated daily plans for each patient on the service and assisted surgical attendings in difficult "cases" (operations) throughout the day. Seniors cared for the complex issues of general surgery patients and assisted attendings with moderately difficult cases. Interns implemented patient plans and assisted attendings with simple cases. Attendings worked on a particular service and operated with the team of residents assigned to that service for the month. Department directors (surgeons themselves) managed administrative issues as-

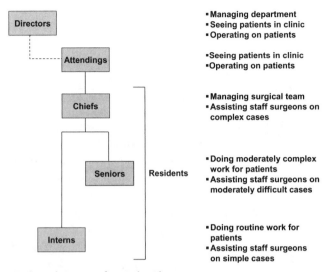

Figure 1.1. Traditional structure of surgical residency programs

sociated with the attendings' activities and the surgical residency program (figure 1.1).

Since residents rotated through different surgical areas such as oncology, GI, vascular, and colorectal as well as working stints at community hospitals, they frequently changed work groups. As an intern, Anne spent four weeks on each rotation, and she had been on the oncology service since Monday. Ryan, who as a senior resident spent six to eight weeks on each rotation, had stayed overnight on call for the service last night.

"Morning. Anything happen last night?" Anne asked. Ryan flipped the lights on, blinking hard once. The call room had no windows and was so small that the one single bed almost filled it. There was just enough room for a bedside table and a walnut-colored wooden desk. A few graying lab coats hung on hooks next to the door. Ryan sat up in his scrubs, picked up his patient printout from the bedside table, and went through the list with Anne. "Anderson, nothing. Whelan, nothing. Cooper, I bolused him [gave him extra fluids]." He went through the rest of the patients. The exchange took about three minutes. Anne took the pile of dog-eared white index cards off the desk—one card for each patient on the service—and shut the door behind her. Ryan went back to sleep.

I had just witnessed the morning version of a long-standing daily work practice—the "signout" between the intern and the on-call resident—a practice that, I had discovered, would have to change if residents were to reduce their work hours to eighty per week. As an intern, Anne was responsible for all the routine work associated with the pre- and post-operative care of patients on the surgical oncology service. Since she had not been on call this night, she had had to stay in the hospital the previous evening until about 10 p.m. to complete this routine work. She then had met with Ryan to "sign out" to him. During signout, she had reviewed general information on the work she had done and alerted him to potential problems. After Anne left, Ryan, as the on-call resident, had taken care of any emergency patient care issues that arose for these patients overnight.

Anne, like other interns I observed before the initiation of the change effort, had not attempted to hand off any routine work tasks (such as completing paperwork required to admit a new patient) during her evening signout. Interns took care of all of this "scutwork" themselves, even though doing so often required them to stay in the hospital until 9 or 10 p.m. and to arrive the next morning at 4 a.m. Historically, signout encounters between interns and residents covering overnight had been characterized by the practice of "no handoffs."

This morning, like most mornings, Anne had returned at 4 a.m. to "pre-round" on all the patients—checking each of them, recording their "vitals" (vital signs), and writing progress notes—before beginning morning rounds with the other residents on the service at 6 a.m. In the morning signout encounter I had just observed, Ryan had signed out to her by reporting on overnight emergencies. Since Ryan, as a senior resident, had not covered routine work tasks overnight, such as gathering vitals for morning rounds, he did not hand off any such tasks to her in the morning signout encounter. Once Ryan had signed out to Anne, he was free to sleep until morning rounds began at 6 a.m.

Anne and I took an elevator up to the eighth floor, and Anne went to the computer on the tall, semicircular desk, "the pod," that wound around the middle of the patient floor. A nurse with a competent air was sitting down inside the desk circle, pencil to her lips, as she read progress notes in a red patient notebook. By 7 a.m., the floor would be full of technicians wheeling hospital carts, nurses talking with one another as they visited patient rooms, and teams of doctors briskly making their rounds. But now, at 4:10 a.m., all was quiet.

Anne stood at the computer on the outside of the desk and sorted the patients on the oncology service in descending order of hospital floors—seventeen patients. Not bad, but she'd be cutting it a bit close if she wanted to be done by 6 a.m. She went to the chipped metal rack outside the pod to find the blue notebook of the first patient on the list—blue notebooks were for recording patient vitals, red were for progress notes. Anne groaned, exasperated. She always had to hunt to find the notebooks, because the nurses never put them back where they should be in the alphabetized rack.[3] One more thing to delay her when she was already pressed for time. Lack of sleep was making her irritable. In real life she wasn't like this. But real life was at least six years in her future at this point.

Anne didn't find looking ahead to be that helpful. She had heard that the second year of surgical residency was also terrible. Third year might be a little better. The lab sounded good (most surgical residents spent two years in the lab learning to do research in the middle of their residency). She couldn't wait to spend time away from here. It made her anxious to look ahead to her fourth and fifth clinical years, because then she would be expected to have reached a certain level of skill.

Anne dug the white index cards out of her lab coat pocket and shuffled through them to find the card for Anderson, the first patient on her list. Her pockets were bulging with pens, patient lists from earlier days, stickers noting the names of the patients she had operated on, a pocket notebook of drugs, and a phone list with consult and department phone numbers. She searched for the red notebook on Anderson and turned to the back of the progress notes to make sure the nurse hadn't made any comments from last night. Nothing. Good. This guy could go home today, as soon as PT (physical therapy) saw him.

She needed to move the patients out so her list didn't get too long. Each patient meant about an hour of work a day. She began to resent people who stayed in the hospital longer than they needed to. When patients got nauseated, she wanted to tell them, "Suck it up." Sometimes she even pushed them out of the hospital sooner than she should have. She knew that was bad. From my observations of the other residents, I knew that this attitude was not unique to Anne. Because they worked such long hours, in order to get through each day residents cut corners on many things not absolutely critical to patient care. Pressing nauseated patients to leave the hospital fell into this category.[4]

Anne went from patient to patient, floor by floor, using the staff-only staircase, finding the patients' blue and red notebooks and writing their vitals on her white cards. She used the list of patients she had printed out to track what she had done on each: L (checked labs), N (wrote progress notes), $ (discharged patient). When she had started her residency the previous July, she had been amazed at the huge amount of hours she had to spend copying numbers from one piece of paper to another. She and her fellow residents had been to medical school at places like Harvard, Stanford, and Johns Hopkins, and she had expected to spend her time during residency operating and engaging in hands-on patient care. If initially all of this paperwork had been useful to her education, it had stopped being so a long time ago. She spent hours each day doing routine administrative work. But she was too tired to worry about that now.

As it got closer to 6 a.m., Anne began to move more quickly, flipping through the notebooks rapidly and taking the stairs two at a time. Mornings were fast-paced because the residents needed to see all of the patients on this list first before showing up in the OR at 7:30 a.m. It was a ritual in surgery to see all the patients in the morning. The residents explained that physicians in other specialties just talked, talked, talked about the patients all day long. Surgeons, they said, always put their hands on their patients and actually took action instead of endlessly talking. That's why you became a surgeon, they explained: you liked the immediate gratification of fixing someone instead of waiting around watching them for ten years and never seeing any improvement.

At 5:57 a.m., Anne finished getting the numbers for the last patient. She took the elevator back up to 8 and went to the pod. Ryan was already there talking to the medical student on the service about Morris, a new patient. With the gallows humor common on surgical wards, they joked about his long list of problems—neutropenia, CNS (central nervous system) dysfunction, port-related infection, pain, nausea, and on and on. Neuro (the neurosurgery department) had turfed him to them (sent him to the surgical ward), and the general surgery residents weren't pleased about it. They hadn't even operated on this guy and now here he was, parked on their service, taking up their valuable time.

At 6 a.m. sharp, Bill, the chief resident, arrived. Anne handed Bill a list of patients. Mission accomplished. At least for now.

8:30 P.M., WEDNESDAY

Anne's day had been relatively uneventful, and because she was the one on call that night, there was no evening signout to observe between her and Bill or Ryan. At 8:30 p.m. I watched her prepare for her night on call. The whole floor had quieted down. There was one nurse sitting at the pod, and the rest were walking around.

At the computer in one of the call rooms, Anne pulled up her list of patients. Only fifteen. That was light. When she had been working on thoracics (the thoracic surgery service), she said, she'd have two sheets single-spaced, and they'd all be complex patients with acute illnesses.

Anne started to prepare some of her discharge orders. As she was doing so, a nurse paged her about a patient who had been operated on that day. Anne went down to the PACU (post anesthesia care unit) on the basement floor to check the patient's wound. She needed to make sure there was no hematoma (subcutaneous bleeding that can occur after surgery). As soon as she returned to the eighth floor, she was paged by a different post-op nurse. She called back curtly, "I was literally just down there." She hung up the phone and turned to me: "Welcome to my world."

She told me that being on call every third night had made her depressed and bitter. Winter was especially bad because she never saw daylight—it was dark in the morning when she came in at 4 a.m. and dark again when she left at 9 or 10 p.m. Anne said she saw her friends about once every three months. She had expected to see them more. It was really hard to be around them. Their table conversation, their perspective, their lives were so very different. Part of her felt irritated listening to it, and part of her asked why she couldn't have it too. She tried not to think about marriage and kids, but she thought about both daily, hourly. "I think it's bullshit. I think about it all the time. I care about my personal life. I don't want to be a woman surgeon, old and alone. I turn a deaf ear, though. You know what it is, so be it."

A patient paged Anne from his home. He had recurrent metastatic colon cancer—a forty-eight-year-old guy with kids. His recurrence was localized, so they had thought they might get the growth out and treat him with chemo. He was young and otherwise quite healthy, a nice person with a family. It was a horrible disease, and right after the operation he had the complication that his bowels didn't start working right away. Now he was leaking gas into his belly. When Anne had seen the leak yesterday, she had hoped that it would go away.

She pursed her lips, upset. I asked her how she handled bad news like this. She said that she tried to be academic about it, that it was to be expected, that this was the way it was. She tried to remember that this was a high-profile tertiary care center—they got the hardest cases, the ones with the most complications, the ones the community hospitals had turned down. But it was tough caring for patients who were so critically ill, she said, especially when she was so tired.

As the night progressed, Anne continued to answer pages. The interns referred to their pagers as "devil machines." Anne's pager beeped, and she took it from her pocket to read the text message. "Can the patient shower?"

"No," she texted back. A few minutes later it beeped again. "Does the patient still need telemetry [connection to a machine that measures data such as blood-oxygen level and sends it to computer screens for nurses to monitor]?" She texted back, "Yes, per order 1 hr ago." She turned to me: "Telemetry is something that is hard for the nurses to do, so they are always trying to get us to stop it."

One problem with the long hours, Anne said, was that she spent a lot of time hating the patients. Sometimes, if they considered her their doctor or if she had made a small difference in their day or their life, it was great. But it was gratifying only briefly, and anyway, it didn't happen a lot. It was hard to build any kind of relationship with them, because she was too busy. She said that she took longer to round in the afternoon than most because she had a sense of guilt. She believed that she needed to give them at least five minutes of her time and not be rushing in, ripping off their dressings, and leaving.

At around 11:30 p.m., Anne went to the call room to sleep. There was one call room for the oncology service; everyone on the team shared it because only one of them was on each night. There were silverfish bugs all over, and no matter how much the hospital cleaners sprayed, they couldn't get rid of them. But Anne was so tired that bugs were the last thing on her mind. She fell asleep right away, praying for no Tylenol calls (routine requests from nurses, preferably handled during the day).

I went down the hall to find a couch in one of the family waiting rooms. Anne said she'd come get me if she got up for anything. She got paged twice overnight. The first page was around 2 a.m. from a nurse who had just arrived at work. Anne had prescribed augmentin, which is penicillin based. The nurse called to check on this because the patient was allergic to penicillin. Anne growled, "Yes I know, dammit, but she's been on it for two weeks with no problem." Then, at 2:30 a.m., she got paged again, this time about Whelan, who had abnormally low blood pressure. She couldn't tell from the nurse's description how bad it was. She got out of bed, swung by the family waiting room to get me, and we went to look at him. There was nothing much to worry about. Within five minutes, we went back to our respective sleeping areas.

3:40 A.M., THURSDAY

My watch alarm went off at 3:40 a.m., and my eyes felt glued shut. I put on my lab coat over my scrubs and went to the supply closet down the hall to look for a toothbrush. Then I went to the cafeteria to get a yogurt and coffee. I had learned that I shouldn't bring food or even coffee to the interns. Interns wouldn't be caught dead eating or drinking during pre-rounding. It went against the valued intern "workhorse" image.

At 4 a.m., I went to find Anne as she pulled herself out of bed to pre-round. By 6 a.m. rounds, two hours later, she was visibly dragging. At this point she had been in the hospital for twenty-six hours straight and still had fifteen hours to go. What exhausted her, she said, wasn't spending a day on call but the cumulative effect of one day of no sleep on top of another. The day before yesterday, she hadn't been on call overnight, but she had been in the hospital from 4 a.m. to 10 p.m. I was exhausted myself, and I obviously hadn't been doing every third-night call for the last year as she had.

During rounds, Bill, the chief, asked Anne whether she had gotten a culture (to test for possible infection) and she hadn't. "Get that," Bill said, curtly. She told me afterward that she couldn't believe she had forgotten to get the culture. She had checked labs and had even written five discharge orders but had totally forgotten to order a culture.

At one point during rounds, Anne fell asleep standing up. Her knees went limp and she fell forward. She jolted awake, looking around quickly to see if anyone had noticed.

She was so tired that she did not write down all the patient plans. After rounds, she looked down her list of patients. She had a few boxes with nothing next to them, and in one of the boxes she had written the patient's name instead of what the task was. She felt she couldn't ask Bill or Ryan what she had forgotten, because she was worried how it might affect her reputation. The hospital was like a fishbowl. Everyone knew what everyone else was doing. So she guessed at what plans to carry out, hoping she was correct. Anne's solution wasn't unusual; the other interns I observed often found themselves in similar situations and handled them the same way.

When rounds ended at 7 a.m., Anne began to order lab tests, put steri-strips on patient wounds, and do the other routine floorwork on her patients. She had a few cases scheduled for later in the day, so she needed to get her scutwork done. "The person post-call always gets good cases," she explained. "It's kind of a reward for staying on after call. It's like, they just took a beating, they were up all night—give them some good cases. It's throwing them a bone."

1:25 P.M., THURSDAY

At 1:25 p.m. we went down to the PACU to get ready for Anne's first case. In the PACU we ran into Bill, who was joking with one of the other chiefs and an attending surgeon. The chief was telling a story about the "train wreck" (patient with multiple, complicated medical problems) he had taken care of the previous night. He described all of the things he had done, and it was clear from the reactions that they were last-ditch efforts. The attending made a motion with his hands showing water going down a drain and a whistling sound to go with it.

The attending left, and Bill and the other chief began to brag about completing a gastric bypass in record time. Attendings at the three hospitals let the residents engage in this kind of banter to create a sense of adventure in what was otherwise a series of long and tedious days of routine operations and endless floorwork.[5] Residents were poorly paid in relation to peers with similar educational backgrounds who worked in other professions. While the annual salaries of residents—ranging from forty-five to sixty-five thousand dollars depending on their institution, state, and year of residency—are comparable to those of professionals in other fields such as nursing or teaching, their per-hour wages were relatively low.[6] Since they worked so many hours, many residents felt entitled to display the traditional surgical resident identity of action-oriented hero; many attendings allowed them this reward to help keep them motivated to work hard.

Anne put on her surgical cap, mask, and booties in the PACU, and I followed suit. Her first case was a breast biopsy. We entered the corridor of operating rooms and went to the scrub sink outside of OR 12. Anne suppressed a yawn as she pumped the soap dispenser and leaned against the metal sink to start the water running. She tipped up her left arm and began scrubbing. She and the medical student talked about the patient, who was thirty-seven. "She is young to have had a mammogram," the medical student noted. "Family history," Anne replied.

The nurses helped us don sterile gowns, and Anne and the medical student prepped and draped the patient. The attending, Dr. Cranford, arrived and they began to operate. The patient had a needle in her breast put there by radiology to mark the spot. Dr. Cranford and Anne would take out the tissue around the needle and send it to radiology; the radiologists would then look at the calcifications and tell them whether they got an acceptable sample of tissue. Dr. Cranford and Anne were on one side of the table. Anne politely asked if she could switch places. Dr. Cranford told Anne what to do and she did it. Then Anne asked whether she could use a certain technique. Dr. Cranford replied: "The tissue is so hard you won't know what is tissue and what is wire. Try it. . . . It looks good. Looks like you are accomplishing it."

As Anne continued, Dr. Cranford said, "Keep that knife down. Go around this way." Dr. Cranford took out the tissue and handed it to the nurse, who marked it with a stitch for radiology purposes. Dr. Cranford was satisfied: "Depending on how much it [the needle] moved between when it was placed and when we started operating, I think we got it. That was a tough one, but you don't get to choose your patients."

4:00 P.M., THURSDAY

Anne assisted Dr. Cranford with a second breast biopsy, and then we went back up to the eighth floor so that she could finish her floorwork before evening rounds. By this point Anne was exhausted and I was on autopilot, but we had at least another five hours to go before we would be leaving the hospital. Anne squinted as she tried to read the handwriting on a white index card next to her computer. Next she put in some new orders to change a patient to PO (oral) meds. She paused a few moments before typing anything. She confessed that there were gaps in her thinking. A few more minutes went by. She appeared to forget what she was doing. She said she needed to avoid sitting in one spot, needed to keep moving.

Anne's exhaustion was not unusual. Many of the residents I followed fell asleep during their workday. And all of them told stories about the places they'd fallen asleep: on a wooden bench in the hall while waiting for the elevator, on a chair next to a patient's bed while talking to the patient in the middle of the night, at a nice restaurant on Main Street mid-conversation on a first date.

Anne told me that she hadn't been on the oncology service before and that the learning curve was very steep. She had done some oncology in medical school and learned the basics but had since forgotten much of it. Now, she said, if she learned things she wouldn't remember them because she was too tired. It was already Thursday, and she wasn't yet where she wanted to be on the oncology learning curve. It was very scary, she said. She had spent her last three days feeling nervous—nervous and scared that she was going to screw up.

But this wasn't as bad as when she had been taking care of the ICU or the ER, where the patients were so sick they couldn't tell you what was wrong. When a patient's condition was really bad, you had to get others to help. But even when emergency or intensive care patients had only minor complaints—say a headache or nausea—you were told to "load the boat," that is, bring in others with more experience, for these might be symptoms of a major stroke or hemorrhage. If you were ever in doubt, you needed to err on the side of calling others in. But you couldn't be calling your chief every minute; you needed to show that you had things under control, and you had to try to pack as much as possible into one phone call.

When she had been on those services, Anne said, she literally would get no sleep when on call—well, perhaps she'd fall asleep for thirty seconds sitting by a patient's bedside, but that was it. She was in perpetual motion. She was so sleep-deprived that she didn't realize what she was doing. She'd take care of all of the acute stuff, she said, but she dropped a lot that wasn't life-threatening. She used to have dreams about missing the most obvious symptoms and would wake up drenched in sweat.

At 4:25 p.m. Anne dozed off again in front of the computer. At 4:40 she jerked her head up and looked around to figure out where she was. She finished copying numbers from the screen onto the index card and put the stack of cards back into the pocket of her lab coat. She rubbed her face, leaned back in the chair at the long, low desk, and said to me, "I'm sure it's ridiculous to look at this from the outside."[7]

Anne left at 9:30 that night.

*　　*　　*

Based on my observations of residents at the three hospitals before the new regulation was announced, Anne's day was not atypical. Since the early 1900s, when William Halsted established the surgical residency program at Johns Hopkins Hospital, surgical residents had traditionally worked 100–120 hours per week. In fact, the term *resident* was coined because these trainees literally were living in hospitals during their training period. Under the traditional regime, even though residents did not officially live in the hospital, they were there for so many hours each week they might as well have been. At Advent, Bayshore, and Calhoun, the long work hours that the highly committed yet exhausted surgical residents worked seemed to have negative consequences both for the patient care they delivered and for their own mental and physical health.[8] But it seemed that things were about to change.

2

Similar Hospitals, Similar Programs

While patients' rights and residents' rights reformers outside of hospitals had long been pressing for work-hours change, the ACGME announcement in spring 2002 that work hours would be regulated starting in July 2003 signaled a new phase in the battle. Before, work-hours regulation had been a threat looming on the horizon; now it was a reality. Directors in surgery at Advent, Bayshore, and Calhoun were under the gun to implement change so that their surgical residents' salaries would be funded and their graduating residents would be allowed to sit for surgical exams.

Subsequent chapters will show how and why change processes at the three hospitals eventually diverged from one another. But part of what makes the story of their later divergence interesting is that the three hospitals were so similar initially—they faced similar environmental pressures, they had similar organizational characteristics and similar top-manager interest in change, and they designed very similar compliance programs to respond to the regulation.

SIMILAR ENVIRONMENTAL PRESSURES FOR CHANGE

In some ways, the environmental pressures for change were fairly weak.[1] While the new work-hours regulation had clear objectives and was backed by the strong threat of loss of accreditation, its enforcement depended on residents' self-reports of weekly work hours. There were many disincentives for residents to report violations. For instance, the identities of those reporting violations were not securely protected, and those who did report violations risked causing their own program to be disaccredited.[2] In addition, sanctions were meted out by the profession rather than the national government.[3] Finally, directors were well aware of New York State hospitals' long-standing use of symbolic compliance; in the past new programs had been introduced to appease external regulators but then not acted upon in daily practice.[4]

In addition to providing relatively weak pressure for change, the environment provided relatively weak frames, identities, and mobilizing structures for internal reformers to use to transform long-standing practices.[5] For example, while external reformers had framed current practices as unsafe for patients and harmful to residents, internal reformers had a vested interest in not admitting that they had inadvertently endangered patient care or that their own education had been in some way deficient. Similarly, the identity of the overtired, overworked resident who was dangerous to patients that the movement had provided to internal reformers, while good for spurring members of the general public to demand reform, was not attractive to residents who would sometimes be working overnight once they joined the profession as staff surgeons. The identity of public advocate opposed to the medical establishment, while useful to external reformers, was not attractive to internal reformers, all of whom hoped to become members of that very establishment. Finally, the mobilizing structures provided by external reformers, such as the reform conferences sponsored by CIR (Committee of Interns and Residents), were not useful to internal reformers who were concerned about the career implications of being seen fraternizing with public crusaders.

Despite the lack of helpful frames, identities, and mobilizing structures, two new political opportunities in the external environment made the traditional system of surgical residency vulnerable to the demands of reformers inside the hospitals—a reduced labor force and an increased diversity in terms of gender and family responsibilities.[6] Historically, surgeons in the United States have occupied a position of very high prestige and pay. In the "glory days" of surgery, directors in teaching hospitals had had the luxury of structuring "pyramid programs," hiring a greater number of surgical residents than they wanted and, over the course of residency, ejecting those whose performance fell short. Despite this harsh weeding-out process, there had traditionally been a greater number of medical school graduates interested in general surgery than intern spots available in general surgery programs.[7]

But recently surgery had become less attractive as a profession. To be sure, with average annual salaries of around $280,000 according to private compensation surveys, surgeons were extremely well paid compared to other professionals, doctors in other countries, and even doctors in other specialties in the United States.[8] In addition to high pay, doctors enjoyed high prestige in society. While the prestige of doctors had dropped somewhat in the past few decades (from 61 percent of respondents rating doctors as having "very great prestige" in 1977 to 50 percent in 2002), it was still extremely high. In 2002, only scientists (at 51 percent) ranked higher.[9] And within the highly esteemed realm of doctors, surgeons were placed by the public at the very top of the prestige ladder.[10]

Despite this high pay and prestige, external commentators believed that the "golden age of doctoring" had passed.[11] This decline was seen to have been caused, in the main, by the corporatization of medicine, the emerging competitive threat from other healthcare workers, changes in the doctor-patient relationship, and the erosion of patient trust.[12]

Within the profession, too, there was a sense that something had been lost. A Calhoun attending, speaking to me late one afternoon in his office, ruminated gloomily on the decline of the profession. "When I went through Harvard Medical School, there were probably 130 people going into surgery every year. Now there are five or ten. They see the writing on the wall. . . . Reimbursement is going down, power is going down." He pointed out that new alternatives to surgery such as endoscopy and interventional radiology meant that patients could be saved without calling in a surgeon.[13] "The need for the surgical white knight isn't as frequent as it used to be." There had been a major attitudinal shift on the part of patients, too. "If I have operated on them on Monday, on Tuesday they want to see me, and part of the stress of medicine and surgery is that Americans are very demanding, not just in their medical care but in everything. They want it all and they want it now, and they don't want to pay for it." Altogether, he concluded, the life of a surgeon was no longer what it has been in the past:

> The personal toll is huge. During residency I did six clinical years. Then I did two years of fellowship, and at the end of those years of general surgery I was on my knees. I was tired. In fellowship, the time demands weren't so high and I was able to eat, to get some sleep, and it helped me a lot. But unless a surgeon has a very supportive home environment, a spouse and family that

are totally behind him, and unless he has his own psychological shit together, it is easy for him to lose it.

And residents were doing more than complaining about the disappearance of the golden age of surgery. They were voting with their feet. Several residents told me a revealing anecdote. A few years before I began my study, one of the hospitals I studied had encouraged surgical residents who were interested in medical administration to go to business school rather than into the research lab during the historical two years off in midresidency. This "business school in place of research lab" program had been initiated, the residents told me, because the directors had thought that business school could be useful training for surgeons who would later take on leadership roles in their departments and hospitals. But, the residents related, the directors had been forced to discontinue this program after several years because all the residents who had gone to business school found greener pastures in the business world and never returned to surgical residency.

In the new, less attractive environment, hospitals across the country had been forced to abandon their "pyramid programs" and replace them with "square programs"—that is, programs that were structured by hiring the number of surgical residents projected to graduate. But even with this square program structure, in 2001, sixty-nine general surgery positions across the country went unfilled.[14]

In addition, demographic changes in medicine had created desires for less grueling work hours among potential recruits. Now more women were training to be physicians. While in the 1970s only 2 percent of surgical residents had been women, by the early 2000s roughly 25 percent of surgical residents were.[15] In addition, more men in training wanted time for family and community life. This increased diversity in the labor force meant that within the three hospitals there were chiefs and senior residents who were disadvantaged by traditional surgical practices. Those practices were well suited to male residents who did not want to take on family and personal life responsibilities, but less so to the new cadre of male residents who, because of new societal expectations, took personal life responsibilities seriously. Changing demographics increased the presence of potential allies inside the hospitals, making it more likely that challenge would be successful.

The pressures of a dwindling supply of surgical residents and their changing demographics were made clear to me when I first met Bob Goodwin, Surgery Department director at Advent. He told me that he was concerned that surgery was no longer attracting the best recruits from medical school.

Bob, in his early fifties, exuded vigor, warmth, and a powerful sense of direction. At six feet one, he had a broad smile and a confident way of speaking that made one believe in what he was saying. When we went to the hospital café to pick up coffee for our noon interview, it was clear that he was also very well liked. He chatted amiably with a nurse as we stood in line at the cashier. On our way out he smiled at a young surgical resident rushing down the hall and said, "You keeping everything in line for us, Allen?" "Yes, sir," the resident assured him.

Once we returned to his sleek, stylish office, he noted that surgery department directors, even in prestigious residency programs, had problems because surgery was becoming a less attractive destination for medical students. Fewer people were applying to be surgeons, and hospitals across the country were not filling their surgical slots. Goodwin explained, "The more I looked into it the more I realized we've got a problem here, and not just a work-hours issue—it's a workforce issue. I began meeting with students, and they told me they really loved surgery, *but* they wouldn't do it because of the quality of life, the abusive environment, the long training periods. And I realized, 'This is for real.'" Over and above the new regulation, the dwindling supply of surgical resident recruits and the increasing percentage of residents who wanted more time for family and community life exerted external pressure for change on all three hospitals.

While the three hospitals faced similar environmental pressures for change overall, there was one area in which the environmental pressures on them varied; however, this cannot explain why Advent accomplished change while Bayshore and Calhoun did not. The hospitals were subjected to slightly different forms of regulatory pressure. In spring 2002, the ACGME announced that the new regulation would go into effect in July 2003. Both Advent and Bayshore underwent additional pressure because the ACGME would be conducting site visits to them;[16] in order to signal their good intentions to the ACGME, both introduced their compliance programs during the residency year of July 2002–June 2003. Meanwhile, since Calhoun was not up for ACGME review until later, its administrators did not introduce a compliance program until the following year, when the regulation actually went into effect.

But this difference in the form of regulatory pressure (ACGME site visit versus regulation officially in place) cannot explain the difference in change outcomes. In 2002, Advent and Bayshore both had impending ACGME site visits, yet only Advent effected change. And Calhoun did not accomplish change during my year there even though the regulation was actually in effect then. One might expect that the environmental pressure that Calhoun faced to reduce work hours (and the risk of loss of accreditation this posed) would be greater in forcing change than would the environmental pressure that Advent and Bayshore faced of a site visit (and the risk of new formal requirements for change this posed) during a time when change was not yet officially mandated. Yet Advent effected change and Calhoun and Bayshore did not. Thus, differences in the form of regulatory pressure cannot explain the difference in outcomes.

SIMILAR ORGANIZATIONAL CHARACTERISTICS

Just as the three hospitals faced similar external pressures, so the organizational characteristics that have been shown to affect institutional change were remarkably similar in all three.[17] Theorists have shown that since larger organizations and public sector organizations are more visible to external constituencies, they are more likely to adopt compliance programs in response to external pressure.[18] Organizations may be influenced by being in the same industry or by being located near other organizations that have already adopted a change.[19] On the other hand, organizations resist pressures to change that require them to act in ways that are inconsistent with their identity and image.[20]

Advent, Bayshore, and Calhoun are similar in all these respects. All three are teaching hospitals associated with major medical schools in the same geographic region. Their residency programs were of similar size; all three hospitals were public sector organizations; and all three had a positive performance history and image (table 2.1).

The structure of authority relations in the three hospitals was also similar. Indeed, before this regulation, the structures of surgical residency programs nationwide—as manifested in roles and relationships among the directors, attendings, and residents—were remarkably consistent. Professional training in surgery followed widely accepted protocols across hospitals, and the work of residents in general surgery was organized similarly. In the professional bureaucracies of hospitals, directors of the surgery department were surgeons who managed administrative issues associated with the activities of the other attendings and the surgical residency program but had little authority over the day-to-day practices of these attendings. Attendings brought revenue to the hospitals by bringing in surgical patients. The attendings both depended on the work of the surgical residents and provided the residents with hands-on training.

TABLE 2.1. A comparison of the three hospitals

	ADVENT	BAYSHORE	CALHOUN
SIMILARITIES			
Location	US urban center in same region	US urban center in same region	US urban center in same region
Size of surgical residency program*	2 directors 23 general surgery attendings 43 surgical residents	2 directors 21 general surgery attendings 41 surgical residents	2 directors 25 general surgery attendings 45 surgical residents
Alignment with public sector	High	High	High
Prior organizational performance	Full accreditation every year for which data are available	Full accreditation every year for which data are available	Full accreditation every year for which data are available
Organization type	Teaching hospital	Teaching hospital	Teaching hospital
Authority relations	Residents subordinate to surgeons	Residents subordinate to surgeons	Residents subordinate to surgeons
Union status	No surgical residents in union	No surgical residents in union	No surgical residents in union
Director background	Career in academic surgery	Career in academic surgery	Career in academic surgery
Resident background	4 years of medical school	4 years of medical school	4 years of medical school
Training period	5 clinical years; 2 lab years	5 clinical years; 2 lab years	5 clinical years; 2 lab years
Work organization	4 teams of residents provide care for approximately 15 patients on a service Tasks assigned according to year of resident Residents rotate onto a new service every 4–8 weeks	3 teams of residents provide care for approximately 15 patients on a service Tasks assigned according to year of resident Residents rotate onto a new service every 4–8 weeks	4 teams of residents provide care for approximately 15 patients on a service Tasks assigned according to year of resident Residents rotate onto a new service every 4–8 weeks

(continued)

TABLE 2.1. (*continued*)

	ADVENT	BAYSHORE	CALHOUN
DIFFERENCES			
Size of hospital**	1.2x beds	x beds	1.4x beds
Resident demographics	77% male, 23% female 63% white, 30% Asian, 7% black 65% general surgery, 35% other specialty	61% male, 39% female 71% white, 27% Asian, 2% black 49% general surgery, 51% other specialty	67% male, 33% female 76% white, 22% Asian, 2% black 73% general surgery, 27% other specialty
Status of residency program	High status: affiliated with elite medical school	Middle status: affiliated with very good medical school	High status: affiliated with elite medical school

* Number of attendings includes attendings on the private general surgery services; number does not include directors. Percentages of female general surgery attendings are 33% for Bayshore, 28% for Calhoun, and 30% for Advent. Numbers of residents and resident demographics do not include clinical residents in postgraduate years not involved in making the change in signout practice on the private general surgery services, and also do not include the non-clinical residents undergoing two years of laboratory training.

** To disguise which hospitals are studied here, actual number of beds is not recorded.

Of course there were differences among the three hospitals—differences in hospital size, in resident demographics, and in the status of the residency programs. But these differences cannot explain why Advent later succeeded in accomplishing change while Bayshore and Calhoun did not.

Take the matter of size. Calhoun is larger than Advent, and Advent is larger than Bayshore. Institutional theorists have suggested that larger organizations are more likely than small ones to adopt compliance programs because they often have greater resources to invest in new programs and are more visible to governance bodies. But all three hospitals adopted similar compliance programs.

Resident demographics at the three hospitals also varied somewhat. Bayshore had a higher percentage of female residents than did Advent and Calhoun and a higher percentage of residents training for one or two years in general surgery before moving on to other specialties. In general, I found female residents and other specialty residents to be more open to the work-hours change than male residents and general surgery residents. One would expect, then, that these demographic differences might make change easier to accomplish at Bayshore than at Advent and Calhoun. But change occurred at Advent, not at Bayshore and Calhoun.

Finally, differences in the status of the residency programs appear to have had little effect. The literature suggests that organizations occupying middle-status positions are more likely to conform to existing norms than are organizations with either high status or low status; organizations with high status have the resources to resist norms while low-status players have little to lose by disobeying them.[21] But there is no clear status pattern in the outcomes. Advent and Calhoun are high-status residency programs, while Bayshore is a middle-status program. But Calhoun and Bayshore resisted change, while Advent embraced it.

In sum, it does not appear that differences in organizational characteristics can explain the difference in outcomes at the three hospitals.

SIMILAR TOP-MANAGER INTERESTS

The three hospitals were also similar in terms of top manager interests. Top managers in organizations have been shown to try to maintain autonomy and control even as they seek legitimacy for their organization. When external pressures run counter to their interests, they may engage in symbolic compliance to varying degrees but often do not embrace change if it diminishes their own power.[22] Top managers may also resist change for a host of other reasons: if it is inconsistent with their training and background, if it doesn't match their experience in other organizations, if it doesn't fit with their professional identity, and so forth.[23] In contrast, if top managers are supportive of reform, they may develop new policies consistent with it, commit important resources to facilitate implementing reform, or even attempt to recruit adherents to reform.[24]

Top-manager characteristics cannot account for the different outcomes at the three hospitals I studied. Directors at all three fought hard to garner resources that would allow them to bring about the change in hours. For example, during an early interview with Bayshore director Robert Beckman in April 2002, he told me that he had strongly lobbied top hospital administrators for resources that would allow him to make changes within his department. Residents worked such long hours, he thought, not because it was necessary for their education but because the hospital wanted doctors who were dedicated and talented—and inexpensive. He understood that implementing the new regulations by reducing resident work hours would be both a cultural and a management challenge, but it was a challenge he obviously relished.

Top administrators at the three hospitals supported the surgery directors in their efforts. One top administrator at Calhoun said: "I think they [the ACGME] are doing the right thing by setting limits [on resident work hours]. We will make it work. It is the right thing, because there are harmful impacts of residency on family life. Also, in the current system, residents have a sense of entitlement after training because of what they have given up to get through. The only way to prevent this is to decrease hours."

SIMILAR COMPLIANCE PROGRAMS

At Advent, Bayshore, and Calhoun, directors planned similar programs to comply with the regulation. At all three hospitals, directors started meeting with the attendings, chief residents, and senior residents several months prior to the new resident year to inform them of the impending regulation and solicit their input about the best way to address it.

I saw the second of these meetings at one of the hospitals. I'd heard from the hospital's directors and residents alike that the first meeting, which had occurred a month earlier, had been both very well attended and quite heated, with surgical attendings angrily defending the traditional system and suggesting that the hospital should try to fight the new regulation. One of the attendings told me that he had pointed out that the public was reacting to a few isolated incidents and did not understand what it took to train surgical residents: "My philosophy is, if it wasn't broke, why fix it? You have one or two isolated stupid incidents, and to make a generalization out of a specific incident is asinine. 'Cause I'll tell you, patients are sicker than they were ten years ago, and in ten years they'll be sicker still, and if you don't have qualified people taking care of them, they're going to die."

Another attending told me that at the meeting he had objected to the fact that outsiders were telling medical professionals what to do: "Part of being a professional is you set your own boundaries and your own rules. Now we've got other people telling us what to do. Right now it's resident work hours, but next it's going to be attending work hours. This happened to airplane pilots, and if we're not careful it will happen to us."

The opponents to reform had apparently gathered momentum quickly, with one after another attending losing their temper as the directors passively looked on. One attending had exploded: "This is all so much bullshit. Who's running that committee [at the ACGME]?"

In the face of this onslaught, the directors had held their ground because they felt that the new work hours regulations were inevitable. As the director of surgery later explained to me: "When Phillip Harris sits in my office today—he is a visiting professor and a traditional good ol' boy general surgeon—and tells me that the ACGME is under the gun from the American Medical Student Association and other groups, and has already made its decision, then we know that regulation is inevitable. We need to find a way to make these changes."

The first meeting had ended in a stalemate, with attendings refusing to support change and directors insisting that a change must happen. The directors called for another meeting, giving notice that "the issue to be discussed would not be whether to change but how to change."

In contrast to the packed first meeting, the second was frequented by only one attending (who arrived halfway through), one incoming chief resident, one senior resident, several low level administrators, and me. We all filed into the conference room in the surgical residency program area a few minutes before 5 p.m., grabbing a Coke and some crackers and cheese from the white formica side table before sitting down.

Tim Williams, surgical residency program director, began the meeting by reminding us that although no legislation mandating a change had as yet been passed, there was every indication that such regulations were forthcoming and that they would resemble the current legislation in New York. Williams, six foot five with a relaxed gait, had a reputation of being cool under pressure and was known as a "surgeon's surgeon"—the highest compliment among surgery insiders. But as I watched Williams in that meeting, I noted that his famous mien of can-do optimism seemed to be eclipsed by an unwonted air of grim resignation. "Last time," Williams said, "we spent the whole meeting discussing if this is a good idea or not, but that is a moot point. When Yale gets put on probation by the ACGME for not abiding by previous ACGME rules, then we know the new regulation is going to happen. So let's try to avoid discussing pros and cons today. We are going to need to have a separate night float team to abide by this new regulation. The question is, how do we best staff it?"

Directors at the other two hospitals held similar meetings to try to get attendings on board with the changes by warning them of the need for new programs to reduce resident work hours either because of impending visits from the ACGME (at Bayshore and Advent) or because of the official start of the new requirements (at Calhoun). But at all three hospitals, the attendings resisted so tenaciously that directors fell back onto working with incoming chief residents. These incoming chiefs would need to manage the day-to-day work on their services in new ways, so they were eager to be involved with designing the logistics of the new staffing programs.

Although attendings at the three hospitals had grumbled loudly about new programs, in the end they saw the writing on the wall. Soon enough they admitted the need to develop new programs, if only to "satisfy the ACGME." As we will see in the next chapter, however, the fact that they accepted a program's formal creation did not mean that they would make a good-faith effort to put it in place to reduce resident work hours.

Once directors at the three hospitals had decided that a new program was required, the directors and incoming chief residents did not spend much time deciding what general form it should take. The obvious solution was a night float program, which added residents to general surgery services to create teams working overnight each night, and which were fairly standard. Such programs had been in place for over a decade in New York State.

Unfortunately, the New York experience offered little concrete evidence to the directors on the best way to accomplish eighty-hour resident work-weeks, nor did it give much of a clue about what impact reducing resident work hours might have on training or patient care.[25] While New York regulations had been in place since 1989, the state had not begun vigorously enforcing them until after 1998. Then, after surprise inspections of a dozen teaching hospitals showed extensive violations of the hour limits, the New York State Department of Health had fined several hospitals and adopted new penalties for nonadherence as part of New York's Health Care Reform Act 2000. And in 2001, the Department of Health had contracted with IPRO (Island Peer Review Organization), an independent, federally financed quality-improvement agency, to conduct periodic surprise visits to monitor duty-hour compliance. Even so, New York State hospitals still had significant levels of violation despite intensive monitoring by IPRO.[26]

In addition to being used frequently in New York, night float teams could often be created with minimal additional cash outlays by taking surgical residents from less busy surgical rotations and reassigning them to the night float team. Hiring new residents was not usually an option for hospitals, because each hospital residency program was funded for only a limited number of residents a year in order to control the number of newly trained surgeons entering the profession. Even had they been able to get approval from the RRC for additional resident positions, directors were loath to do so, concerned that this would dilute the educational experience of the existing residents by decreasing their caseload.

So using New York's night float team as a model, the directors at all three hospitals worked with incoming chief residents to design the new programs. Incoming chiefs had a better feel than did directors for how busy each existing rotation was. They helped to determine which rotations could be cut most easily so that their surgical residents would be freed up to serve on night float teams covering general surgery services.

To staff these teams, in some cases residents were taken from quite busy rotations. For example, all three hospitals chose to eliminate a community hospital rotation in order to free up a resident for the night float team. Obviously, this had negative consequences for care providers at the community hospitals, who now needed to find a way to accomplish work that had been previously done by a surgical resident. However, faced with tough choices, the directors and incoming chiefs chose to reassign residents allocated to other departments rather than to pay for new senior physicians out of their general surgical budget. In addition to reassigning residents, directors and incoming chiefs in all three hospitals decided to hire several PAs to help with administrative work during the day.

Once incoming chiefs told them where to best reassign residents and place PAs, directors secured the resources for the night float programs and PAs by negotiating with hospital top managers. They also notified department directors outside of general surgery that they would be eliminating some of the existing surgical resident rotations. Dr. Beckman, program director at Bayshore, noted that top management support was necessary for this because "people in these other areas don't like it when you tell them you're going to take away their surgical resident."

In order to understand the change processes that later unfolded at the three hospitals, it is critical to understand the structure of these night float programs in some detail. Historically, chiefs and seniors had worked approximately 100 hours and interns approximately 120 hours per week. Under the new system, night float programs would allow residents at all levels to reduce their hours by 20 per week by virtually eliminating nights spent on call. This would put chiefs and seniors in compliance with the regulation. To further reduce intern hours to about 80 per week, interns would need to reduce the number of hours they worked on a regular workday from roughly 17 (4 a.m. to 9 p.m.) to roughly 13 (6 a.m. to 7 p.m.) by handing off routine work to night float members in signout encounters.

This would require residents to change a long-standing daily work practice—"signout"—between the intern and the resident covering overnight, described in chapter 1. To recap, historically surgical interns had been responsible for all the routine work associated with pre- and post-operative care. When interns were not working on call overnight, they met with the on-call resident to "sign out" by reviewing general information on the work done that day and alerting the on-call resident to very sick patients. The on-call resident took care of any emergencies that arose overnight. But according to the residents (and consistent with my observations prior to the introduction of the night float programs), interns did not attempt to hand off any routine work tasks, such as completing paperwork required to admit a new patient, to the resident covering overnight. Interns took care of all of this "scutwork," even though doing so required them to stay in the hospital until about 9 p.m. and arrive the next morning at 4 a.m. to gather data on patients before morning rounds began at 6 a.m. At 4 a.m., when the intern arrived, the resident who had stayed overnight on call would sign out by reporting on any overnight emergencies. Since the on-call resident had not covered routine work tasks such as gathering "vitals" (patient data) for morning rounds, he or she did not hand off work tasks to interns in morning signout.

Under the new system at the three hospitals, interns would be required to hand off routine work to more senior residents in signout encounters. The new program, following the New York model, would add three surgical residents to the private general surgery services, creating a "night float team" to work overnight. Position 1 would assist with highly complex patient care work such as surgical emergencies; the position 1 resident would not interact with interns. Positions 2 and 3 would cover both simple and moderately complex patient care work and routine administrative work overnight; these residents would interact with the interns working during the day. Positions 2 and 3 would be staffed by either a designated resident, who would work six nights a week for an entire rotation, or a rotating group of surgical residents, each of whom would work overnight once or twice a week and leave the hospital the following morning.

Day interns at the three hospitals would be expected to hand off any of their work not completed by 6 p.m. to the position 2 and 3 night float members. These night floats would cover all simple and moderately complex patient care and routine work from 6 p.m. to 6 a.m. and hand off any uncompleted tasks to day interns. Residents would work thirteen-hour days, six days per week, to allow for one hour of overlap on each end of the day. These work-hours reductions would not entail a reduction in income for any residents; annual salaries were fixed.

One might have expected that the plans for the new night float programs would have been greeted with exultation by the residents, who would be dramatically reducing their workweek with no corresponding reduction in pay. But many residents did not rejoice. In fact, they did the opposite.

*   *   *

While the change trajectories at the three hospitals would later diverge from one another, the hospitals initially faced similar environmental pressures, had similar organizational characteristics, and had similar top-manager interests for change. With the announcement of new ACGME regulations, directors and incoming chief residents at the three hospitals drew on the New York State model to develop similar compliance programs. Yet despite the external pressures for change and the creation of the new programs, many at the three hospitals initially resisted work-hours reform. In the next chapter I explain why.

3

Meet the Iron Men

Tahir Azim, an incoming chief resident at Calhoun, was vehemently opposed to the impending work-hours change. When I interviewed him in early June in the Calhoun surgical resident lounge, it was clear that even bringing up the topic angered him. "The problem," he spat, "is that these rules are being made by people who don't know the first thing about surgery."

Tahir was from New York. His uncle was a surgeon, his father was an oncologist, and his mother was a nurse. When he was eight years old, he had seen a movie of open-heart surgery. When he saw the surgeons stop and then restart the heart, he knew he wanted to be a surgeon when he grew up.

Tahir had gotten married five months before he started at Calhoun, and he and his wife had had a baby in his third year of residency. Tahir told me that he often went two to three days without seeing his son awake at home. He noted that it was hard for his wife to have any semblance of a normal life with him because of his schedule.

But, he said, he was still "old school" when it came to work hours. His philosophy was that this was the life he had chosen. He felt that he was a good father, not a typical father who was home for dinner every night, true, but still a good father who enjoyed the time he had with his son as precious.

And he found it galling that no one in charge of making the new rules had bothered to ask the residents what they wanted in all of this.

Tahir was not alone in feeling this way. In fact, the mandated reduction in resident work hours was resisted by many within the three hospitals. The attendings uniformly balked at the changes, some more vehemently than others. Their resistance is perhaps not surprising. They feared the changes would increase their workload, since the residents they depended on for help would be working fewer hours. They worried, too, that they would need to communicate with a greater number of people about patient care. Late one afternoon at Advent as we waited in the PACU (postanesthesia care unit) for the next case, an attending openly spoke to me about his worries:

> Now I won't be able to trust that they're [the residents are] going to get done. They'll probably get done. But I'll have to double-check everything, because I'm the one who's ultimately responsible for these patients. They'll have to leave after their eighty hours. . . . I'm going to be doing my most acute cases, be it trauma, middle-of-the-night disaster, or what, and I'll be trying to figure out who the *fuck* to call, because the intern signed out to this night float person and my chief resident's gone.

More puzzling was the response of some of the residents, who resisted change and condemned those who tried to attempt it. On the face of it, reform would seem to benefit them by reducing their work hours. But many of the chief residents were concerned that the change would force them to rely on a greater number of residents rather than their own interns to do routine work, and both chiefs and senior residents thought they would be required to take on some of the routine work traditionally done by interns, who would now be in the hospital for fewer hours.

As I talked to the attendings and many of the chief and senior residents at the three hospitals, I sensed that the strength of their negative reactions was far out of proportion to such small adjustments in surgical practice. Particularly for chiefs and seniors, taking on a bit of routine work would seem a small price to pay for dramatically reducing their own work hours. And after all, the chiefs already were communicating regularly with their senior residents as well as with interns, so logistical costs of the change appeared to be minor. Moreover, chiefs and seniors who would take on more routine work would now be well rested, since they would no longer be working overnight every third night on call.

What wasn't there to like?

In this chapter I explain why a change aimed at providing greater patient safety and improved quality of work and personal life for the residents was resisted by many at the three hospitals. The intensity of their alarm suggested that defenders of the status quo were not making decisions only on the basis of their material interests; they were also drawing on their taken-for-granted beliefs, their feelings about appropriate and inappropriate conduct, and their understandings of behavior appropriate to their position.

THE INSTITUTIONAL CONTEXT OF SURGICAL RESIDENCY

The proposed work-hours changes presented a challenge to the very core of American surgery—to its closely held values about what it meant to be a surgeon, its long-standing authority relations that privileged some doctors over others, and its fundamental beliefs about the best ways to care for patients and educate residents.[1] Because of such widespread and deeply ingrained principles, attendings and many chiefs and senior residents at all three hospitals fiercely resisted the new regulation.

American surgeons and surgical residents have traditionally described themselves, and have been seen by others in and outside of the hospital, as action-oriented male heroes who singlehandedly perform death-defying feats, courageously acting with certainty in all situations.[2] This social identity of the heroic surgeon originated in the early history of the profession, when surgery was performed amid perilous circumstances and lives were saved despite horrendous hygienic conditions. It has been perpetuated in contemporary times.[3]

Authority relations in surgery are aligned with this professional identity.[4] Tasks and responsibilities are rigidly prescribed by position: the chief residents lead the team, and the interns occupy the lowest rung on the ladder. The beliefs supporting this professional identity and authority relations are "continuity of care" for patients (best patient care is achieved when one surgical resident takes total responsibility for a patient from the time of surgery to the time he or she leaves the hospital), "learning by doing" (residents must learn surgery through hands-on experience), and "living the life of a surgeon" (surgeons must always put their patients first, over and above any personal commitments they may have).

One way in which US surgical residents have traditionally lived up to this culturally shaped ideal is by avoiding handoffs. The taboo on handoffs in surgery originated in the 1890s, when the director of surgery at Johns

Hopkins, William Halsted, developed programs meant to mold residents in accordance with this professional identity.[5] Since Halsted's time, surgeons have occupied a high position in the status hierarchy of the medical profession and in society as a whole. Surgery's high status has been built and maintained in part by long work hours, a macho demeanor, deference to seniority, and avoidance of handoffs between residents.[6]

Everyday practical understandings of these surgical principles—valued roles, long-standing authority relations, and legitimating accounts—shaped the residents' behavior inside the hospitals I studied. These principles afforded residents an appreciation for the demeanor of a surgical resident in good standing, that of an "Iron Man." They allowed residents to allocate resources and authority according to their position in the strict surgical hierarchy. And they provided residents with particular justifications for this prescribed demeanor and deference structure. An Iron Man identity and a strict hierarchy were seen as necessary to achieving good patient care and good resident education.[7]

While all residents were aware of professional dictates, most residents did not act according to them in all situations. In fact, many lived in a state of some tension with the Iron Man image. In the next chapter I will describe how several categories of residents excluded from the Iron Man club questioned surgical institutions and, as a result, played a crucial role in the change effort. But first it is necessary to understand the traditional surgical culture and to see how those whose behavior complied most closely with traditional prescriptions were afforded the highest status inside the hospitals.

VALUED ROLES

Everyday understandings at the hospitals specified three valued surgical resident roles—interns, seniors, and chiefs—and a narrative of prescribed actions appropriate to these specific roles. In the social world of surgical residency, the standard narrative was for residents to come in as interns who "don't know anything" and to be "molded" by those more senior to them so that seven years later they could act as chiefs.

Interns (first-year residents) were expected to act as "workhorses" who could be counted on to do whatever their chiefs asked of them. According to their prescribed role, interns arrived at the hospital at 4 a.m. and left at 9 or 10 p.m. They were expected always to be on time for rounds, to stand up rather than sit when entering orders (putting orders into the computer for pre- or post-operative patient care), to enter these orders at machine-gun speed, to rush quickly in and out of patient rooms to collect data (rarely conversing with patients), and to "live for the OR." These interns were taught to answer back rapidly when they were being mercilessly "gunned" by their chiefs during "teaching" on afternoon rounds; answering something, anything, was better than showing trepidation or doubt.

"Strong" interns were expected to take ownership of their patient data and never to hand off their work to anyone or sign out their pagers to other residents when they did leave the hospital. In the idealized narrative, interns accomplished every task on their list by afternoon rounds without help from others. A revered attending at Advent explained the characteristics of a good intern to me one day while we scrubbed for surgery:

> As an intern you are the workhorse of the team. The beast of burden. First one there and last to leave. . . . Like Bill Cronin from last year. He was from Detroit and hadn't gone to an Ivy League school. He was a hardworking SOB who had worked as a car mechanic. He never had anything given to him on a silver platter. You'd give him a huge scut list, and he'd roll up his sleeves and say "I can do it." Not "Why do I have to be the one to do it?"

Good interns took "real responsibility" for their patients. "As an intern you felt like 'I am that patient's doctor,'" one senior explained. "I was with them when they got admitted, and I will be with them when they get discharged. I'm not going to leave their side. I'm going to round on them twice a day at least." Strong interns were the ones others saw as "burning the midnight oil" and "walking out of here at 10 at night." They were willing to do whatever it took to get the job done. One attending summed up the ideal of the perfect intern:

> The best intern is the one who hasn't gotten off of the treadmill of life—has gone right from high school to college to med school to residency. If they've had a great life, it's hard for them to go from that and give it all up and go back into the system. Versus if you haven't ever done anything and have nothing to compare it to. At the rank meetings [meetings where residents are chosen], they throw the picture up, and if they show that someone is forty-four years old and a world-famous chess player who spent summers teaching Tibetan monks primary care and now he has the realization he wants to go into sur-

gery, it is a problem. If you take someone who has been coddled and told they are the best and the brightest and who has achieved a lot, and he is thrown in a pool with the lowest common denominator and viewed as a mule rather than a great genius, then it will be a problem. At 3 in the morning, when the patient is vomiting all over and you have to put in an NG tube and draw blood, it doesn't matter if you were on the cover of *Time* last month. You may have outside interests, you may be this or that. But the bottom line is you need to get the work done.

Iron Man chiefs (fifth-year residents), by contrast, saw themselves as "dogs of war," as "the biggest, baddest SOBs around, beating up on the meddies [medical residents] and beating up on the radiologists." They were "commanders" in charge of molding new interns. One of the junior attendings perfectly described the cultural ideal for a chief one day during lunch. He talked about how he had acted on morning rounds when he was a chief:

I was someone who was very focused on rounds. One guy used to take around his little mug of coffee when he rounded. And we were like "What the fuck are you doing?" I finished at 7 a.m. with my rounds. I hated finishing at 7:30 because that's when the OR starts. I think it's important to break bread with the guys all the time. So you finish at 7, team breakfast. Then you sit back, buh, buh, buh, the game last night, joke around, have your coffee, bust each other's balls. But from 6 to 7 it's game face, boom, no chitchat, no extraneous conversation, just give me the data.

I was incredibly demanding that they know their patients. If they were like "I'm sorry I didn't have a chance to see all of these patients," I'd say, "*Stop.* OK, we're rounding at 5:30 am tomorrow," and then the occasional 4 a.m. ones. So the interns had to show up at 1 a.m. to get the numbers, you know, having gone home at 10 p.m. Or I rounded late. At 4 in the afternoon I went home and then came back in at 8 p.m., just so those guys stayed late and realized that you know what, you guys can't leave but I'm gonna leave. I'm gonna leave, and I'm gonna go home, and I'm gonna come back when all the data's done.

But I looked out for them. When interns were on for Iron Man weekends [Saturday morning through Monday night], I came in on Sunday morning and grabbed their beeper for four or five hours just so they could go home, shower, pick up the mail, see the wife, and then come back. I also told them when they did a good job, because you have to give them that little carrot. If it's all stick, you can't motivate people. Like the slot machine, intermittent re-inforcement. It's a lot of stick. It's a lot of stick early on, but then you lighten up, because once they're trained, once you break their will and you've molded them, then there's less stick.

As part of molding the interns, chief residents were expected to act as drill sergeants, to aggressively shame the interns by yelling at them in front of an audience. Residents termed this "giving a beating." One attending said of this practice:

> Some chief residents have a difficult time trying to control their interns or trying to mold them. In other words, they can't break their will. I never had that problem [smiles]. I think it's a problem when chiefs are afraid to break people's will. It's like Marine Corps boot camp. You break everyone's will and then you mold them in your image. And if some bucking bronco comes in, day one, you need to do it fast. Ideally you don't start off with a huge thing, you just say, "All right, this is the way to do it." But if they continue to do it, then it's public dressing down. It does work.

Iron Man seniors (second-, third-, and fourth-year residents) saw them-selves as "wingmen." They were there to support their chief in enemy ter-ritory. Seniors had responsibility for neither the running of the service (which the chiefs did) nor the care of individual patients (which the interns did). But they were expected to protect their chiefs by working alongside them, "watching their backs" and "taking one for the team" when neces-sary. As wingmen, seniors made their chief more capable by providing help where necessary. They were alert to potentially dangerous patient situa-tions, treated these patients before problems occurred, and kept the chief informed about them. They were also expected to tell stories that made the chief look good. And they took the less interesting cases so the chief could get better operating experiences. When necessary, they attacked enemies—attendings in other specialties outside of surgery, nurses, lab technicians, or other members of the hospital staff.

While some actions were prescribed for particular roles, others tran-scended all roles. For example, no matter what their rank, "strong" resi-dents were expected to be men, "Iron Men." They were also expected to go into general surgery rather than other specialties, to focus single-mindedly on work, and to act "individualistically" by "trusting no one" and by "living in the hospital."

An Iron Man was a "go-to guy" with "nerves of steel" who was "unflappable" under pressure. Iron Men could be counted on to "make it happen" no matter what the circumstances. Iron Men were also tough enough to work longer hours than any other resident in the hospital: "Pain is just weakness leaving the body." One resident told me that he always made sure to shave and look neat because he wanted to show his chief that no matter how much the chief beat on him, he would never break him. In addition to looking sharp in their scrubs, surgical residents were expected not to need either food or sleep. One PA said, "Don't let them fool you. It's not that they don't have enough time to go get something to eat. It's that they don't want to be caught sitting down there in the cafeteria." Junior residents I followed often sneaked off to call rooms to "catch a few Zs" midmorning after their night on call, but they "definitely didn't advertise it." One of the interns I followed showed me his dog-eared copy of the standard surgical textbook *Advanced Surgical Recall*, which summarized perfectly the surgical residents' view of sleep:

> *Sleep Deprivation:* The best offense to combat sleep deprivation is to be in good physical shape and to be motivated. Staying up for 48 hours is no different than participating in a ultramarathon. Many residents find they benefit from caffeine, orange juice, hot showers, brushing their teeth, doing push-ups, running steps, yelling, changing their socks, or listening to loud music. Studies have shown that sleep deprivation is mainly a mental problem and that physical abilities remain intact until extreme deprivation of sleep occurs. Try not to sit down, because sitting is conducive to falling asleep quickly. Overall, it is an attitude: "I am hardcore and I need no sleep!"[8]

As part of the Iron Man persona, residents were expected to follow a cultural vernacular of macho: short haircuts, tucked-in scrubs worn low on the hips, green surgical caps and masks around necks long after leaving the OR, fast striding movements during morning rounds and cocky swaggers in the evenings. The "best" Iron Man stories revolved around the game last night, "smoking" (hot) interns, "house calls," (late-night visits to girlfriends), and call-room exploits. Here is a conversation that took place between two residents in the surgical lounge one night on call as they told war stories about one of their favorite chiefs:

DANIEL: Before we'd start rounds every day, we'd have to get an update from Jim. He'd have a different woman every night. One night it was some Danish chick wearing a white lace thong and taking a house call from him. The next night it was a redheaded Irish waitress. He'd come in and say, "Thank God I'm on call. I need to rest." [Laughter]

RYAN: Yeah, when he was on call and I was the intern, he used to say, "After 11 you can always come get me. But it is a sign of weakness. I don't want you to come knocking on my door."

Other Iron Man stories involved partying and breaking rules designed for the general public. One night on call, an attending told this story of a legendary chief from the days of the giants:

Bob McKenna was the guy. He was a wild man. When he was working he'd work like a dog, but when he was off, he was an unbelievable partier, unbelievable. Did you ever hear the story about the end-of-year party at the Ritz? We always used to have the party at the Westin, and then when Pierce [director] came, he wanted something a little flashier and wanted to go to the Ritz. So we had the first couple at the Ritz, until Bob decided to trash the Ritz Hotel.

In the old days, the graduating chiefs would chip in money and get a suite and they'd go up after the party and drink and basically invite everybody up. So after the party that year they all went up to the room and Bob was totally shit-faced and being loud and obnoxious, and the whole room was loud and obnoxious. About sixty people up there playing poker and smoking cigars. And there's a knock on the door and it's the manager: "You know, we've had some complaints from people on the floor." And Bob is totally shit-faced and he's got a bottle of Jack Daniels and he yells in the guy's face, "Shut the fuck up, we'll be as loud as we want."

So the manager asks him to leave, they call security up, and coming out Bob throws the Jack Daniels bottle and it crashes into the chandelier of the Ritz. Bob then starts tussling with the security guy, he breaks free, and he tries to go through these double doors. He opens the double doors and there's like a thousand balloons for a wedding the next day, and they all get released. So now there are balloons all over the lobby and security is bullshit. They throw him out of the hotel and he drops his pants and takes a leak.

So I guess they gave Pierce some huge bill, and he's reading it and he's like "A thousand balloons, I don't remember any balloons." And then they basically said, "You're not welcome anymore."

Part of being an Iron Man was being action-oriented and daring, an orientation embodied in the traditional sayings surgical residents tossed back and forth: "Often wrong, but never in doubt." "If you wanna make an omelet, you gotta break some eggs." "Everyone makes mistakes—that's why it's a seven-year program." "Don't let the skin get between you and the diagnosis." "The only prescription this patient needs is hot lights and cold steel." "It's showtime." "Giddyup." "Got it covered." "Fire it up and *bring it on*."

As well as enacting the macho role, Iron Men were expected to take individual responsibility for their patients. One saying I heard over and over from Iron Men was "Trust no one, expect nothing, suspect sabotage." Taking individual responsibility meant never handing off work to anyone and never signing out pagers. Residents were expected to avoid the help of PAs and to discount the input of nurses and other physicians when making their decisions. One attending said: "You do everything there is to take care of that patient, and you do it yourself. You don't expect anyone else to do it for you. You need to know what makes patients tick, what their likes and dislikes are, what their allergies are, and what medications they're on."

Finally, Iron Men prided themselves on "living in the hospital." Their "fellow residents," they boasted, "were their family." Joe Curry, a Bayshore attending, told me one evening in the PACU as we waited for his operation to begin that when he had done his residency it was an every-other-night program, with no concern about how many hours one worked or whether one had been home to see his family or his own bed. And Joe had the battle wounds to prove it. He said that he divorced his first wife when it became clear that she wanted the benefits of being a surgeon's wife without the costs. Joe's confession was not unusual. The attendings and residents constantly told stories with bravado about breaking commitments with disaffected wives and significant others, who more often than not were blamed for having chosen to have relationships with surgeons: "Just because you want to be in the circus doesn't mean you like cleaning up after the elephants." Another attending told similar tales:

> Residency is legendary for breaking up marriages. They say that Wallace [a prior department chair] only took married men because they had a stable home life and hot meals waiting for them at home. And he only took single women because he was not worried about them getting pregnant. Everyone loves to celebrate [elite teaching hospital] as a hardcore program because they say that they had a 110 percent divorce rate. Guys would come in married, get divorced, get remarried, and get divorced again before their seven years were up. . . . It was not uncommon for guys to burn out their marriages early on. If they did stay married, their wives had to put up with a lot. One of

the guys in my year entered the program when his wife was pregnant. And they wouldn't even give him the afternoon off after the delivery. So his wife had to take a taxi home.

Family obligations always took second place. About parenting, one of the residents said, "Have your baby here — at least you'll get to see it for the first few days of life." An attending told me that when he was a junior resident, he was not allowed to go to his grandmother's funeral:

> I'll never forget the reaction from the chief. He was like "She's not going to know if you're there or not."
>
> [What did your family say?]
>
> My family just sort of understood. I said, "I'll try, but I don't think there's any way I'm going to be able to go."
>
> [Did the hospital need you?]
>
> Absolutely not. That was about "You are a surgeon first and your personal life comes second. And right now we need you to pull chest tubes and do this and that." And you're like "You fuckin asshole, I hate you, blah, blah, blah." But you're too tired to let that grudge hold, because they are beating on you about something else. And they also instilled in you that you wouldn't want to do that to your fellow residents who are going to be holding the fort down.

LONG-STANDING AUTHORITY RELATIONS

Just as valued roles prescribed how good residents were expected to act, so long-standing authority relations provided surgical residents with an understanding of their position relative to others, a sense of their social place and the power, status, and privilege that came with it. These authority relations specified a particular hierarchy of privilege of senior residents over junior residents and surgeons over other medical providers.

Some of the prescriptions for enacting positional relations of seniors over juniors involved appropriate dress. In each hospital, the dress for seniors versus juniors varied in ways that were subtle but well recognized by insiders. In one of the hospitals, for example, residents in their first through fourth years were expected to wear a short white lab coat with the hospital name embroidered on the top left pocket. In contrast, the chiefs were expected to wear a long white lab coat with their full name embroidered on the pocket. Differences in dress were indicators of positions of privilege relative to others and of the rewards that awaited those who respected traditional power relations.

As part of this dress, "good interns" at all three hospitals always seemed to display at least two pens in their top left pocket. This was, I was told, to heed the maxim "There are two types of interns—those who write things down and those who forget." But it was also to signal to more senior residents that they were ready to take any orders the seniors might impart.

Work activities also reflected relative positions in the hierarchy. "Pre-ops" (checking patient charts prior to surgery) and "admits" (admitting new patients), for instance, were labeled "scutwork." Doing this kind of scutwork, residents said, insulted the dignity of a senior resident.[9]

There were other displays of deference that were prescribed. Juniors were expected to "know their place" and "pay their dues." They were not to "whine." Deference appeared in exchanges between chiefs and interns over patient plans. One intern noted to me: "As a chief you don't want to hear arguments. 'Maybe my idea is better' does not fit into the hierarchy." Another intern said the same thing, more bluntly: "If the chief wanted my opinion, he'd beat it out of me." One chief described his interactions with an intern this way: "Out at Riverview [a community hospital], Sue Radan was my intern. And I barked at her. She put up a lot of lip. Like 'In my opinion the patient should get a CT scan.' So I barked: 'Surgery is not a democracy, it's a dictatorship! I don't care about your opinion. Seven years from now, you can give your opinion. Your job now is to do what I say and to keep your mouth shut.'"

In the culturally accepted Iron Man narrative, if juniors "paid their dues," they could rise in status over time. One attending who had come up through the residency program reminisced: "People can get disillusioned in the first few years because they don't want to spend their days doing discharge summaries and drawing blood. The reason you stick with it in the early years is that you look up to see the chief residents on top of the hill and you think, 'I want to be like them.' I was like 'I am your putty. Take me. Mold me. Make me great.'"

As well as promising rewards for good behavior, the accepted narrative threatened punishment for those who strayed from the traditional path. Seniors reinforced their demand for conformity by regularly meeting any complaints from juniors with taunts of weakness. "Cry me a river," they would respond to a junior's complaint. One of my favorites, overheard as a chief responded to an intern: "Do you want some cheese with that whine?" What was occurring, of course, was that the seniors taught the juniors how to act in accepted and time-honored ways. Not to do so could have dire consequences.

Just as long-standing authority relations placed seniors over juniors, so they placed surgeons above both the general public and other kinds of medical doctors. One nurse told me that a prior thoracic surgery department director had a framed picture of Michelangelo's Creation of Adam in his office. When people asked him about it, he'd tell them that God was the first thoracic surgeon.

Similarly, in surgery, "back in the day" stories emphasized the rewards that lay in store for those who persevered through the years of long hours in surgical residency. In every profession, stories of the glory days provide members with tales of heroes and villains, mastery and blunder, and victory and defeat that serve as both motivators and warnings to aspiring members about how to act. While such stories were part of the everyday fodder of surgical conversations, few I met had a greater stock of tales about the days of the giants than Jack McLaughlin. Jack was a gruff young attending of Irish heritage with tightly cropped copper hair who had recently come up through the Advent residency program.

I had arranged to follow Jack one night on call. When I paged him to meet up with him, he told me to meet him and Daniel Cohen, one of the senior residents, at The Grill, an upscale steakhouse. When I arrived, Jack and Daniel were sitting at the bar, joking with the bartender, who knew them by name. They were halfway through dinner—24-ounce porterhouses. Daniel had a Guinness, and Jack was drinking ice water since he was on call. Jack began to tell a story about how he had decided to become a surgeon.

He had grown up in Pennsylvania with an older sister and a younger brother. No one in his family was a doctor. His parents ran a diner. But his high-school biology teacher made science fun and interesting, so as an undergraduate at Carnegie Mellon, he took the whole pre-med regimen: physics, biology, organic chemistry. He went to medical school at Dartmouth.

As a third-year medical student, he thought he wanted to become a general practitioner. Surgery was the last thing he wanted to do. "In med school, people who wanted to go into surgery were gunners, cutthroat. They'd go to class in scrubs even when not in the hospital."

Jack had his first day in surgery in that third year. It was cardiac surgery. Up to that point, all of his medical rotations had started at 8 a.m. The chief of cardiac told him they would begin rounding at 6 a.m. Jack smiled as he told the story to Daniel and me:

The chief was a former marine. He was the toughest SOB I had ever met. He showed up on rounds screaming at everyone. I was like "Who the fuck is this guy?" My first case was at 4 p.m., a redo, redo mitral valve aortic valve [third operation on the same patient because prior operations had not been effective]. At 3 in the morning we were still in the OR. I contaminated the attending surgeon [violated sterile technique] three times during the case. And finally, at 3:30 in the morning the patient arrested and died. The attending surgeon stormed out and the cardiac fellow left, saying, "Close 'im up." So there I was with a dead guy on the table with an open chest. The scrub nurse hands me the suture and says, "Hurry up. We need to get out of here." I didn't know how to tie knots or anything. So I ended up sewing this guy up with a bow on his chest. I was like "These guys are assholes." I told my roommate, "If I ever tell you I want to do surgery, stop me." I crashed at 4:30 a.m. and ten minutes later my alarm went off. And it was like that for six weeks.

Despite this harsh initiation, Jack decided to follow up with a six-week general surgery rotation:

It was great. I loved the team. I was on with one of my good friends. I had a great chief resident and a great 3rd year. They'd go out for drinks afterward. They had the same sense of humor I had. A lot of the medicine people were snotty and stuffy and wanted to go home and read the latest New England Journal of Medicine.

Then he had to decide if he really liked surgery, so he took a year off to do surgical research:

I didn't want to make a career decision on a six-week rotation. Training was seven years, every other night, no family, no anything. On my surgery rotation, I worked so hard but I was so pumped. I loved the operations. And surgery is something where you can have dramatic and immediate impact on someone's life. On medicine I didn't work as hard, but I was tired all the time because I was bored. So I did five surgical sub-I's [subinternships]. I didn't want to commit to seven years based on six weeks.

Jack's account was typical of the ones I heard from many attendings and residents. Choosing surgery hadn't been an easy decision. They knew that it would change their lives. But they loved it so much, they really had no other choice—the bright lights of the operating room, the challenge of the anatomy, the drama of life and death.

And like other stories of choosing surgery that I heard, Jack's story made it clear that he had made this life-changing choice based on more than a love for the technical challenge of surgery or the ability to make a difference in the lives of patients. Jack continued:

> During my research year, I worked in an animal lab run by an attending surgeon. The surgeons were unbelievably fun guys. They'd take the sailboat out. My mentor would drive me into New York with a case of wine in the back. They worked hard and partied hard. I was like "This is fun." They treated me so well. "This is the greatest thing since sliced bread." I got to present at a conference in London.
>
> I asked them, "Where do I go to be the best surgeon I can be?" Advent had a great reputation as the place to go and get trained and come out the other end as an unbelievable surgeon. Now it is less of a boot camp. It used to pride itself on that. Thompson was the chief of surgery, and the residency was like the Thompson club. Surgery ran the hospital. If a surgery resident had a fight with an ER resident, as long as you didn't punch 'im, you were fine. Thompson would call you into his office and you'd say, "I was just trying to take good care of your patient, sir." And he'd say, "You didn't hit 'im, did you?" "No, sir." "Argh, OK, I back you 100 percent."
>
> The chiefs used to have prayer meetings with the boss. They called 'em prayer meetings because Thompson was like "Argh, who's the troublemaker this time?"
>
> It was more of a pyramid structure then. There were always stories about residents working for four or five years and then being cut loose and needing to find new places to go. The thing was that hospitals needed more help at junior level than at senior level. We would lose two people a year. You wanted to survive. The few. The chosen. The proud. You wanted to be the one to come out the other side.

As Jack told his tale, he clarified for his audience—in this case Daniel and me—why it was worth it for residents to respect the rigid authority relations in surgery. On the one hand, by attending to minute differences in status, residents were reinforcing hierarchy among the underlings within surgery.[10] On the other hand, they were living up to an image more broadly. By choosing surgery, residents were choosing more than just a particular

specialty with a particular form of work. They were also choosing a professional identity—heroic, aggressive, confident, decisive, work hard–play
hard. And what went along with this identity was an elite status position
at the very top of the medical hierarchy. Jack's story suggested that no one
messed with the surgeons. And if they tried to, the surgeons ruthlessly
crushed them with little fear of retribution. Jack portrayed their power in
the hospital as absolute, even godlike. Residents who respected the surgical
hierarchy, it seemed, would receive their just rewards.

LEGITIMATING ACCOUNTS

Roles and authority relations in surgery were part of a highly articulated system of interpretations that the residents used to make sense of their social
world.[11] Yet the demands of a strong hierarchical system, long work hours,
and a macho identity created strains and contradictions for the residents.
Members of all professions develop accounts to deal with difficulties when
questions are raised about the worth of the group's activities.[12]

   Within the surgical social world, residents needed to be conscious of and
manage the physical and emotional strain generated by the long hours they
worked, the unquestioning obedience expected of them, and the necessity
to be "strong." They did this in part by developing collective accounts of
their world that interpreted the working of long hours, deference to seniority, and machismo as normal rather than strange. Three key legitimating
accounts provided residents with justifications for the social order of which
they were a part. I call these accounts "ensuring continuity of care," "learning by doing," and "living the life of a surgeon."

   A strong belief in "continuity of care" supported traditional roles and
authority relations.[13] Attendings and residents at all three hospitals said
that they realized the public was skeptical about the wisdom of working
long hours, but the public simply did not understand that reducing resident
work hours actually would be detrimental to patient safety because it would
interrupt the continuity of care. This, they said, would lead to an increase
rather than a decrease in the number of patient errors. Iron Man attendings and residents believed deeply that handoffs between team members
were more detrimental to patient care than were fatigued surgeons. One
day early on, I naively asked an attending in between patients on a clinic
day why 100–120 hour workweeks were so sacred. Exasperatedly, he explained that handoffs between residents were detrimental to continuity of
care: "You need to treat everyone like you are taking care of your mother.

That patient's care could very well depend on how anal you are about find-ing out what their allergies are, what medications they're on. You need to know every detail, and you need to do everything yourself. Because when there are a lot of handoffs . . . stuff falls through the cracks and things get missed."

In addition to distrusting handoffs, many of the surgical attendings and residents vehemently denied that being tired was harmful to their patient care. No matter how tired they were, they felt, when they got under the lights in the OR in an emergency situation, they were able to focus well and operate effectively. "All this talk about being tired is such bullshit," one attending asserted. "When you get a code trauma and you've been up all weekend, the adrenaline starts to flow and you get your game face on. You are like that until you know the situation is under control." Another chief made the same claim:

> We have these Iron Man weekends. You're on call from Friday morning to Monday night. But you are never tired. You are never tired when it is im-portant. I have yet to fall asleep while someone is coding. I have slept at the bedside of many an ICU patient, and the nurses come and wake me up and say, "These are the latest lab values." I wake up, look at them, and say, "OK, this is what I want to do," and then go right back to sleep. But I never feel like my judgment is impaired, like "Oh my God, these numbers mean nothing to me."

As a justification for long hours, "continuity of care" was tightly linked to the cultural persona of Iron Man and the strict hierarchy in surgery. In order for residents to provide continuity of care, they had to be "tough" enough to work very long hours. And in order to provide this continuity of care, residents believed they needed to work longer hours than the at-tendings—a belief that supported the hierarchy. While attendings were ul-timately responsible for the continuity, hierarchy relations prescribed that it was the residents who must remain in the hospital late to check CT scans or admit new patients or order lab tests, and arrive early to check patients' progress overnight. The interns were expected to work the longest hours because they managed the day-to-day work on the floor for these patients and therefore they had the most detailed knowledge of the patients' prog-ress and plans.

If the "continuity of care" account related to patient care, the "learn-ing by doing" account related to resident training. "Learning by doing" was seen by Iron Men as necessary if residents were to become skilled at the important things in surgery—in their view, developing dexterity in the form of "good hands" and cultivating a sense of "what is going on with a patient." In order to learn surgery, the account suggested, residents must garner a practical and tangible sense of "knowing how to handle things."[14] Residents learned best to make decisions alone and under pressure, Iron Men said, when they worked under the stressful conditions of their training.

One attending emphasized the importance of gaining hands-on skill and "street smarts" versus "book smarts." Over coffee in the cafeteria during a slow night on call, he elaborated:

> Surgery is a body contact sport. . . . There are certain people who, if I had to retake my recertification exam [for the American Board of Surgery], I would definitely have them take it for me. But would I have those same people operate on a loved one? Absolutely not. Surgery's difficult even though you may know the moves to do. Like, I'm looking at a patient with this process and this disease. They need this operation. But between the brain and the hands there's a disconnect. We say, "Often wrong, but never in doubt." I may not know what's going on, but I'll be able to get in there and figure it out afterwards. There are certain people who are very slick surgically and very good, but do they score 99 percent on their boards? No. But they are damn good doctors, and they are very compassionate and they do what's best and safe for the patient.

Similarly, a resident with Iron Man stripes emphasized the importance of a junior resident learning by doing under the tutelage of a senior resident: "You learn by being here. There is a huge amount of information passed on in an ad hoc fashion at 2 o' clock in the morning when the senior resident and you are trying to get the pressure up or the IV in. You need to be the one managing it, doing it, in order to learn." Among the Iron Men, conventional wisdom was that learning the valuable skills necessary for being an attending required spending as many hours in the hospital as possible during residency.

Iron Men had many ways of defending their views. One of the most persuasive was provided by an attending in a late-night chat in the PACU:

> There is a reason for why it has been that way for a hundred years. If it's your mother, you don't want your surgeon saying, "You know, Mrs. Smith, I've never seen this before," or "I'm not as adept as I could be at doing this opera-

tion, but I'm really well rested." Like when you are getting on a plane, you don't want to hear the captain say, "Buckle your seat belts. I haven't flown as many times as I should have up until now, but I've had a great lifestyle." You learn so much more by doing cases and being by the bedside when a patient is sick.

Frequent nights alone on call were seen by the Iron Men to be crucial for resident learning. One evening as I followed an intern overnight on call, he told me: "The nights you get blasted on call make you learn. You have to get it done because no one else is there." He then told me a story about the first time he had made a decision to intubate. It was only his fifth night on call in his first rotation as an intern. He was working at a community hospital and watching a patient in the ICU. The patient wasn't doing well, so he ordered a blood gas test. The patient had more than normal CO_2 levels in her blood and was having difficulty breathing. He had never intubated anyone before except in a controlled environment when the patient was under anesthesia. His chief was twenty minutes away. The ER attending was the only backup in the hospital. The intern called his chief and told him that the chief needed to come in. His chief told him to get the stuff set up and call the ER. The chief added, "If it needs to happen before I get there, just do it yourself."

The intern sighed as he told me that he didn't end up having to do it himself. But he needed to make all the decisions—when it was time to intubate, when to call the chief, what tests to order. The story ended when the chief told him that he had done some things well, some badly. "You should have done this and that. Do it next time." The intern ended the story with a frequently heard surgical mantra: "So it's a constant trial by fire. You need to call them to let them know what you've done, but you have to choose to give this drug before you call them. It is a good way to learn. . . . The mistakes you make you never forget. And you'd never make mistakes that would truly hurt the patient." The "learning by doing" account justified the long hours Iron Men spent at work. It also reinforced the hierarchy of the apprenticeship relationship created between knowledgeable seniors and inexperienced juniors.

The final account that supported surgical residency's traditional long work hours was "living the life of a surgeon." Iron men attendings and residents constantly told me that surgeons needed to have a single-minded focus in order to learn surgery. They had to learn to do surgery when they were tired. And this was altogether consistent with putting patients first.

Thus, they needed to work long hours now so they could embrace the tough lifestyle required of a surgical attending later. Highlighting the importance of a single-minded focus to me one night in the resident lounge, an Iron Man senior explained:

> The problem comes in the fundamental belief: either you are here to learn to be a surgeon or you are learning to be a surgeon while life is going on. I believe the former. Surgery shouldn't be part of what you do. It should be all of what you do.

An attending noted why residents needed to learn to operate when tired:

> There's a lot of stress and pressure as an attending. You need to be up on call all night, and operate the next day. And that's a learned skill. If they don't learn it now, how are they going to do it later?

Finally, on working long hours, an attending defended the practice in the following way:

> We're going to give them [the residents] a false idea of what it means to be a surgeon if they work only 80 hours. I'm worried that people will think that working 80 hours is what they will do afterwards. On a weekend like this one, I work Friday morning through Monday night. That's 110 hours right there. I do 90 straight hours on call and then go into a full day Monday and a full week. . . . And if they work more than 80 hours now, then it will be easier for them to accept 80 later. They will have something to look forward to.

This hypothesized need for "living the life of a surgeon" during residency helps account for the Iron Man's macho demeanor and long hours and for residents' ready willingness to work harder than attendings.

THE INSTITUTIONALIZED PRACTICE OF NO HANDOFFS

For any given situation they found themselves in, residents drew on their shared understandings of these valued roles, long-standing authority relations, and legitimating accounts to decide how to act. These surgical institutions provided residents with a repertoire of morally appropriate actions associated with problems encountered regularly and an account for why these behaviors were appropriate.

Reducing work hours would require changing practices in signout encounters; this, in turn, would force residents to violate some of their most cherished roles, authority relations, and beliefs. In the prestigious *New England Journal of Medicine*, an attending summed up the significance of the signout encounter: "Signout . . . [is the] daily transfer of patients from one medical team to another. . . . In the medical units of hospitals, hundreds of such exchanges happen every week. . . . [This] transition is, perhaps, the most controversial legacy of ACGME's mandate. The scheduling contortions are just minor nuisances. The real challenge of the 80-hour workweek is that it . . . contorts the idea of residency itself."[15]

In the traditional world of surgery, residents knew how, when, and where to engage in signouts. Basically, surgical residents were to avoid handoffs. Residents at all three hospitals knew that this was the appropriate practice. By staying until 9 or 10 p.m. to complete all the routine work on the service, interns played the culturally appropriate "beast of burden" role of beginner who was tough enough to withstand long hours, trusted no one, and lived in the hospital. By not handing off work to the resident on call, they showed deference to their seniors. And by remaining in the hospital as much as possible, they felt they were offering the patients the best care and learning as much as possible.

LIFE AS AN IRON MAN

Only by understanding the valued sense of self the Iron Men possessed, the long-accepted hierarchy relations within the profession, and their beliefs about the best way to deliver patient care and educate residents can we understand their patterns of behavior. Even so, I found myself wondering, early on, whether all their sacrifices were worth it. As I continued my fieldwork, I came to appreciate the rewards for those who could endure the ordeal of surgical residency. For the attendings and many of the chief and senior residents at the three hospitals, the sacrifices of acting like an Iron Man were justified in part by what they would gain when they made it to the top of the surgical hierarchy. These rewards became clear to me one morning as I followed Matt Baker, a fourth-year surgical resident soon to be a chief resident at Advent.

Six foot two, with a black goatee and green surgical scrubs worn low on his hips, Matt looked a quintessential Iron Man. At 7:30 a.m., as he walked into the OR for his first case, Matt went up to Sherrie, a sixty-year-old OR nurse who had been working in the Advent OR for thirty years. His green eyes alight with mischief, Matt said: "Excuse me, ma'am, I'm going to be the resident on this case; I'm Matt Baker." Sherrie beamed as she gave him a big hug. "Where've you been! And where has Paul been?" Matt said he'd call Paul (another incoming chief resident) for her right now. He dialed Paul on his cell phone and, winking at Sherrie, handed it to her. She said, "This is Sherrie calling from OR 12 with Matt Baker. We're having some trouble, and we need you down here right away." Sherrie smiled as Paul joked that he would be right down.

Matt had just returned from several rotations away from Advent. This morning was like a homecoming for him. Everywhere he went, female nurses, young and old, smiled broadly at him, cheerfully welcomed him back, and quickly carried out whatever orders he gave. Patients effusively thanked him, attendings good-naturedly joked with him, and junior residents listened respectfully as he told tales of surgical cases mastered and patient emergencies averted due to his skillful operating during rotations away. Watching Matt made me realize how he and many others at the top of the surgical hierarchy were both extremely powerful in the hospital (and in society at large) and seemingly loved by everyone, respected by everyone. They were treated like heroes. They had paid their dues, had endured, and were now on top of the world.

INSTITUTIONAL CONTRADICTIONS

Once we understand the sense of professionalism and the high status that attendings and residents achieved by complying with the prescriptions of surgical institutions, it is much easier to understand their resistance to the new regulation. Still, an outside observer would be likely to note that while understanding such institutions makes residents' initially puzzling behaviors comprehensible, there seem to be countless inconsistencies in their views and practices. For example, governing oneself by the saying "Often wrong, but never in doubt" promoted decisiveness in the face of uncertainty and stress, but it certainly was not in line with evidence-based medicine. Obeying the tenet "Trust no one, expect nothing, suspect sabotage" bolstered a strong ego and a belief in one's own efficacy, but it undermined the teamwork that is often necessary in surgery and discouraged contributions by other providers with specialized expertise. Wearing scrubs outside the hospital allowed exhausted residents to save time during their extremely busy days but hardly contributed to sterility in the OR. And swaggering around the hospital and bragging about their "house calls" allowed male residents to garner high status with Iron Man peers but had nothing to do with accomplishing good patient care.

Institutional theorists have noted that it is just such internal contradictions that provide space for institutional change to occur.[16] Role prescriptions such as acting decisively in the face of incomplete information may be well suited to one situation (for example, when a patient with multiple complications requires emergency surgery) but less effective in another (for example, when a patient with multiple complications requires a less time-sensitive operation). Authority relations such as those that require attendings to act as "dictators" may have been appropriate at one time, when patient care outcomes depended on a single surgeon's operating skill, but are less functional today when patient care outcomes depend on the effective collaboration of a clinical team. And institutions that work well for one set of actors (for example, male residents with wives at home to care for children, shop for food, prepare meals, and take care of housework) may not work well for a different set of actors (for example, male residents with wives employed outside the home or female residents without partners willing to take care of all of their personal life responsibilities).[17] Such institutional contradictions provide a source of tension and conflict that can reshape the consciousness of actors and spur them to attempt to transform existing arrangements.

*   *   *

Everyday practical understandings of surgical principles shaped the residents' behavior inside the hospitals. Valued roles afforded them an appreciation of the appropriate demeanor of a surgical resident in good standing, that of an "Iron Man." Long-standing authority relations allowed them to allocate resources and authority according to their position in the strict surgical hierarchy. Legitimating accounts provided them with justifications for this prescribed demeanor and deference structure. Because doing so would have violated these surgical institutions, Iron Men like Matt, Jack, and Tahir would never have dreamed of supporting reduced resident work hours.

But at the three hospitals, not all the residents were as comfortable in and supportive of the Iron Man culture as these three. I soon discovered that although all the residents I followed recognized the rules of the culture and could, either eagerly or reluctantly, act in line with them, many residents questioned traditional surgical understandings. The motives of those who questioned, of course, varied, but they were out to change longstanding practices and, if necessary, take on those who defended surgical institutions. These internal reformers are the subject of the next chapter.

4

Potential Reformers

Once we understand the institutional context of surgical residency, the interesting question becomes not why so many residents resisted the seemingly small changes in practice required by the new regulation but why any resident would want to embrace change. After all, the high status and identity possessed by the attendings and many of the residents was so inextricably intertwined with the Iron Man ideal that the new regulations could not seemingly be seen as anything other than threatening to their very sense of self.

But the Iron Man ideal was quite literally beyond the reach of some residents. As social movement theorists have noted, power imbalances are imported into the workplace from society at large, and members with disadvantaged social identities in the world outside often receive fewer rewards and opportunities for training and promotion inside organizations than do their more privileged counterparts. These members of subordinated groups are likely to become internal advocates for reform.[1] I saw this dynamic at work in the three hospitals I observed. Because of their disadvantaged social identities, some residents were assumed to have no right to claim the Iron Man ideal. They were excluded from certain spaces, and they were not allowed to use certain language, wear certain clothes, express certain emotions, or engage in certain tasks that belonged to the high-status Iron Man role.[2]

In this chapter I will describe the residents at the three hospitals who became internal reformers. They came from four groups: incoming interns who did not yet understand the rules of the surgical social world; residents for whom general surgery was not their ultimate career path; female residents; and male residents who wanted to take on more personal responsibilities outside the hospital, who were uncomfortable with the macho Iron Man persona, or who were particularly patient-centered.[3]

INCOMING INTERNS

I talked to most of the incoming interns at the three hospitals before they started their residency training. To a person, they were supportive of the new regulation. Like new members in any profession, they were ignorant of traditional practices, the accounts that justified these practices, and the roles that imparted moral value to them.[4] While they did not yet understand the surgical social world, they were quite familiar with the arguments that had been made by the patients' rights and residents' rights reformers, and thought they made sense. To them, working 80 hours per week rather than 120 sounded like a good idea.

OTHER-SPECIALTY RESIDENTS

A second group of internal reformers at the three hospitals was composed of residents who were transients in surgery. These were residents in non–general surgical specialties such as urology, ophthalmology, emergency medicine, or pathology. They were training in general surgery for only one or occasionally two years before moving on to their primary specialty.

These "other-specialty" residents (my term)[5] were disadvantaged in the surgical social system because many surgical attendings, chiefs, senior residents did not want to invest time in training them. As one Bayshore chief said bluntly, "Why take time to instill responsibility when these interns aren't ours? When you get a general surgery intern, you lean on them more, teach them more. But these guys are just warm bodies."

Nor did attendings, chiefs, and seniors give other-specialty residents the same opportunity to "live for the OR" as they did the general surgery residents. Chiefs routinely assigned better cases to the general surgery residents and invited them to "scrub in" to witness particularly interesting cases. "I try to be pretty good about case assignment," one chief insisted. "If one of those guys [other-specialty residents] is doing a good job for me on the floor,

I'll reward him with good cases." But he went on to confess, "I definitely save the most interesting ones for the general surgery residents. They're the ones who really need the experience. Internship year is a time where they learn things that will stick with them for the rest of their career."

Other-specialty residents were usually not assigned to as many general surgery rotations as were their general surgery counterparts, so they were often not aware of daily routines on the floor or the acceptable behaviors that defined these routines. Chief residents often publicly shamed other-specialty residents for not acting according to the norms of general surgery. Consider the following episode of a public shaming. I quote from my field notes at some length because this episode illustrates not only how other-specialty residents in the three hospitals were treated but also how Iron Men enforced compliance with surgical institutions:

Jim Diaz, an ER intern, had just been assigned to his first general surgery rotation. Typically, the service was covered by one chief, one senior, and one intern, but because there were so many patients on the service, Jim had been assigned to "float" as a second intern. I followed Jim during his first morning. At 6 a.m., he entered the surgical pod for morning rounds. Everyone else on the service—the chief, the senior, and the general surgery intern—was already there. Jim didn't know that juniors in surgery, as a sign of respect for their chief, always arrived before the chief.

Rick Wong (an Iron Man chief) was sitting at the pod desk. Everyone else was standing respectfully on the other side of the pod. Wong, a stern figure in his starched white lab coat and short military haircut, scowled as he scanned the list. Morning rounds started with "paper rounds," where the intern told the chief about patients on the service before the team went to visit each patient in person. Wong quickly started reading off patients' names from the top of the list. The patients for whom Jim was responsible were those at the top of the list.

"McKinnon?" Wong called.

The previous night, Jim had been handed eleven white index cards by the floating intern whom he was replacing on the service, one for each patient Jim would be taking care of. Each card included all the vital statistics and test results for a particular patient, written in an order that was standard for the general surgery residents. Jim paged through his cards for McKinnon's, but before he could find it, Wong began to rapidly read details from the white sheet of paper that Felipe, the other intern on the service, had given him. "98.2, 101, 160 over 90, 9.5, 1.7 . . ." By his brusque manner, Wong made it clear he had expected Jim to be giving him this information, not the other way around. Surgical interns were expected to present patients by reading numbers in the same order at all rounds—average temperature, high temperature, blood pressure, calcium level, magnesium level, white blood cell count, ins and outs (fluids taken in by the patient and expelled)—and then to rapidly give their recommended plan of treatment. Even if Jim had found McKinnon's card before Wong lost his patience, Jim wouldn't have known what he was to say and in what order. He was new to general surgery and had never participated in this particular ritual before.

"CT scan showed left peritoneal fluid collection," Wong continued. "She needs an ostomy consult and metabolic support for TPN. What meds is she on?" Jim read from the card. Wong asked another question. Jim hesitated. He didn't know the answer. Mike, the third-year resident, jumped in. "She has a transvenous pacer on her right side."

"Anything on her left?" Wong asked. "No? So skip the right side, left IJ." He curtly fired off instructions: he wanted all the numbers and he wanted them *fast*. "She's on all her pre-op meds?"

"Correct," Jim answered.

"Do blood cultures on her. What were her labs yesterday?"

Jim read them. Wong wrote them on his patient list.

Wong rushed ahead to the next patient on the list, "Widman?"

Jim flipped through his white cards, frantically looking for the vitals but not finding them.

"What was his last coag?" Wong asked, his impatience continuing to show.

Jim, flustered, began to read a number, then stopped abruptly. "Sorry, this is the wrong card."

As the rounds went on, Jim tried his best to use the previous intern's cards for the first time, but he kept making mistakes. Wong went for the jugular.

"Callahan. What was the CBC on her? Do you have it or not?"

"No."

"Get the CBC on her," Wong said curtly. "Listen carefully to everything I say. Freeman. What meds is he on?" He began tapping his foot. Jim looked at the card, squinting. "I can't read the writing. Sorry."

"OK, redo all of your cards. This is unacceptable."

Next, Felipe, the general surgery intern on the team, presented his patients, briskly reading all the numbers on each in the standard order. "Smith: "98, 101, 130 over 80. Passing gas, belly non-tender, clears today and home tomorrow." Wong nodded in agreement.

Wong finished these paper rounds by asking about Terrell, the last patient on the list. Then he grabbed his papers, and the rest rushed down the staff-only staircase trying to keep up with him. Wong went down the stairs so fast that he swung on the end of each handrail to make the turn. He needed to be in the OR by 7:30, and had to see all of the patients on this list first.

The first patient was McKinnon. All four team members went into the room and stood around the patient's bed. Wong said, "I'm Dr. Wong, Dr. Umberto's chief resident." Now that he was in front of a patient, his curt manner had disappeared. He was very friendly and smiling. "OK, you're doing great," he said placidly. "Any questions?"

The team walked rapidly on to the door of the next patient—Widman. "How are you doing? I'm Dr. Wong, Dr. Lin's chief resident." He prodded the patient's stomach. "Does that hurt? OK, someone from the medical service will come see you. We still don't think you need surgery. Did you get up and walk yesterday? Good."

The team spent about two minutes with each patient. After they left Widman's room, Wong asked Jim whether anything had grown in Widman's culture. "I don't know," Jim replied. Wong moved his hand down abruptly from his shoulder to his hip to emphasize his anger. He spoke in a low, clipped voice: "Check-these-twice-a-day."

At 7:15 a.m. they saw the last patient, Terrell. As they left the room, Wong barked, "Five o'clock rounds." Jim, disconsolate about his first encounter with his new chief resident, sighed heavily as he walked to the nearest computer and, resignedly, began to enter orders.

Like the rest of the other-specialty residents I observed, Jim was treated as a second-class citizen by Iron Men attendings, chiefs, and seniors. Other-specialty residents often did not know the rules and had to learn them the hard way. Because the attendings and chiefs did not see these interns as "their own," they were unwilling to take the time to teach them.

Perhaps not surprisingly, all the other-specialty residents I talked to supported work-hours changes. These residents composed a large percentage of the residents at the three hospitals (37 percent). As we will see later, they played an important role in the reform movement. Less invested in surgical roles, authority relations, and justifying accounts than the general surgical residents, they were outsiders who supported change.

FEMALE GENERAL SURGERY RESIDENTS

Many of the female residents at the three hospitals also advocated reform. Female residents occupied inferior positions on the surgical wards, though perhaps it was not as readily noticeable as it was for the other-specialty residents. In fact, when I began observing the female residents, my first impression was that they lived up to the surgical ideal. I was struck by how "macho" they acted. Like the male residents, many of them told stories of idiotic medical residents, unflappable attendings, annoying nurses, and "train-wreck" patients (patients with multiple, complex medical problems). They strode rather than walked during morning rounds. They accomplished everything on the scut lists on their own, paged jokes back and forth with other residents, and lobbied their chief residents for more difficult cases.

Yet in time I realized that even though they often acted like Iron Men, they never completely lived up to the Iron Man expectations in the eyes of the male attendings and residents. One female senior at Calhoun told me:

> One of our sayings is "Sometimes wrong, never in doubt." If you say that, it projects a certain confidence, a very overt, leadership, Calhoun personality. But it's impossible for women to act like that. And I think that if you try, you're not rewarded for it. . . . I think the people who are in charge—I don't think it's in their conceptual framework that a woman can fit the role they have, because the role they have in mind is specifically male. The residents I work with every day think I'm competent. My chief said to me yesterday in the OR, "I think you're very advanced. You can operate better than your level." But in the attendings' minds, in their feedback to me this year, I'm not confident enough. I don't go around acting like I already know everything, because I think I have tons of stuff to learn, and it's a huge field, and that's why it's a seven-year residency. But that ends up being seen as a lack of confidence. One of the attendings told me that he's worried that I won't be a good leader.

Many of the female residents also felt that they could not get away with acting in the same ways as the male residents. Another female senior explained:

> There is something in surgery where the chief or attending keeps asking questions until the person gets it wrong. We call it pimping. At some point

they are satisfied even if the person can't answer the next question. But it's not only about finding out if the person knows the answer. It's also a way of asserting dominance. You never see female residents aggressively pimping the way male residents do.

There were other differences between female and male residents. Male residents were permitted to explode, to lose their tempers and scream at more junior residents in front of an audience. In fact, aggressively shaming residents in this way was an important part of the commander pose of the chief residents. Chiefs were expected to "break the will" of the interns by loading on work and then berating them in front of others if they failed to complete everything on their scut list. I never observed a female resident act like this. The one female resident who occasionally used a harsh tone of voice was described by others—men and women—as "a bitch."

Male residents were also allowed to use language that female residents were not. Although female residents were permitted to swear (and the female residents I followed swore a lot), they were not allowed to tell highly graphic jokes about male and female anatomy. Male attendings and residents also censored themselves around female residents. As one female resident put it: "The guys, especially the attendings, don't feel comfortable joking around with me in the same way. The residents know who you are better. So they let you into the world they are in. But there is still stuff they won't say in front of you." A male intern indirectly confirmed these norms on the floor by telling me how the tone and atmosphere changed when there were no female residents on a particular rotation. Without the women around, he said, "we could just let loose and not worry about what we said."

Female residents were also limited by where they could go in the hospital. For example, a favorite pastime of male residents at all three hospitals was "appreciating" women. This involved going to the front lobby of the hospital in the late afternoon to check out women going by. It also involved "making rounds" on good-looking new nurses. If a male resident met a new nurse or physical therapist who he felt was attractive, he'd page his male friends to make rounds on her floor. This behavior was an important element in performing the Iron Man image.

Two other important ways to act out the Iron Man persona were working out at the gym and going drinking. Women were, by and large, excluded from these activities. One female resident noted: "A lot of these guys joke around with the surgeons, go running with them, go out to dinner and drinking with them. No staff surgeon has ever asked me to go running. . . . We end up missing out on a lot of the interaction with the staff surgeons, and on the learning that comes with it."

Many of the female residents also felt that other hospital staff did not give them the support that male residents received, support that implicitly bolstered the Iron Man persona. Nurses at all three hospitals, I was told, assiduously helped male residents, but they were less helpful to female residents. One described an incident where she said she became so upset that she grabbed a phone away from a nurse: "It's so frustrating. These nurses will do anything for the guys. The guys just have to smile at them and they bend over backwards to help the guys out. But for me, they won't even follow my written orders. They question me and sometimes I just do it myself instead of going through the hassle. I got into a fight with one of the nurses because she had ignored my orders and the patient almost coded [died] as a result."

In addition to occupying an inferior position in the surgical social world, many of the female residents had trouble fulfilling expectations in the multiple social worlds of which they were a part. Tensions most often arose because of a discrepancy between how they were expected to act as surgical residents and how they were expected to act as women outside the hospital. One female senior at Bayshore talked about how hard it was to be a "good girlfriend" while being a surgical resident:

> I'm so tired all the time. If I am not talking or doing something with my hands, I'm asleep in two minutes. . . . My boyfriend asks where I want to go to dinner. "I dunno." "What movie should we see?" "I dunno." It doesn't matter because I'm just going to sleep through it. He's thirty-five and isn't sure he wants to wait for kids. I couldn't have children during residency. I wouldn't want to do that to a kid. I want to be done with residency. . . . The guys here have it a lot easier. Women are more accepting of a husband off in another place. Like, "My husband is a surgeon, he is out saving lives, and I need to stand behind him. It's OK, honey, I'll take care of the laundry, because you're doing more important stuff."

Some female residents found the two roles—the Iron Man resident who lives in the hospital and the wife and mother who lives outside—utterly incompatible. One senior female resident was so reticent to reveal her "other life" to those in the hospital that she was in the program for several years before anyone knew that she had a child. She said she had been told by a prior female chief resident that she should never tell anyone because it would hurt her reputation as a surgical resident.

One morning before the new night float programs were introduced, I followed intern Karen Battista on morning rounds. The morning is worth recounting because it illustrates some of the challenges faced by female residents at the three hospitals.

Karen wore the standard green scrubs, enlivened by a silver necklace with a large turquoise star. Despite this feminine touch, I was struck, as I often was when following the female residents, by how much Karen acted like "one of the guys." As the intern on the team, Karen was in charge of leading the team from one patient room to the next. Striding quickly from room to room, she paused briefly outside each one to rapidly fire off the expected string of numbers. Once inside, she briskly got to work taking down bandages and pulling NG tubes, with barely a nod to the patient.

Like her male counterparts, while Karen was forceful and serious while reporting her patient plans, she slipped easily into surgical resident razzing whenever the occasion presented itself. During rounds, John, another intern, passed us. Karen smiled and made a point of looking down at her watch and then back up at him, mocking him for having committed the cardinal sin of sleeping through his morning rounds the previous week. At the end of rounds, Karen played the macho resident game of lobbying Will, the chief, for a more difficult case: "You don't want that gastrectomy, do ya, Will? How about throwing something my way?"

But once Will and the other members of the team headed off to the OR, Karen's macho, "make it happen" manner disappeared. She told me how she had almost "jumped off of a cliff" the day before: "I went to a case, scrubbed in, and the attending didn't even recognize me. He thought I was some nursing student! After being here almost a whole year! I like to think that the guy interns and I are all in it together, but something like this hammers it home that we are very different."

Perhaps, Karen thought, the attending didn't recognize her because she had been wearing the same "shower cap" that the nurses wore. While all surgical residents wore green scrubs and white coats, male residents wore a particular kind of surgical cap in the OR, like the ones worn by male surgeons on TV. In contrast, female residents at her hospital wore surgical caps that looked like and indeed were called "shower caps."

Still, Karen was angry. She had worked 120 hours a week as an intern for almost a full year, and an attending had not recognized her. Karen confessed that she couldn't stand being left out of the boys' club. She hated to admit it, she said, but one of the main things she had liked about surgery from the beginning was that it was so macho. Her first summer in med school, she had gone to work for an internal medicine doctor in a small town in Arizona.

> At Arizona, there was a certain type of surgical personality. It was a ton of fun. The people were laid back but intense. Intense jokers. Interesting to be around. I liked the guys and the good-ol'-boy hardcore surgeons. They were the most edgy, the most interesting. Everything was intense. When I came here, they spent a lot of time sizing up what kind of girl I was. How much I could take? They poke you and see how you respond. Like, will I use the word *fuck* and not have some reaction when they do? They realized that I don't care. It didn't take them very long. They know they can tell whatever around me. But the more senior people won't do it. They refuse to tell me certain things. The other residents know what I am like and what they can say and can't say. But take one step outside and they will treat you like a foreign woman.

While Karen talked about the problems she faced as not being quite "one of the guys" in the hospital, another big problem, she said, was finding a guy outside who would put up with her schedule:

> I've only had one date since I've been here, and I had to cancel it to work late. It looks to me like all of my friends' lives have progressed and mine hasn't. I'm frozen in time, I'm on a treadmill, and my friends have moved on. Being a surgeon isn't so great as a woman. These guys can go out and meet anyone anywhere who will date them. . . . It is a huge asset for men. It means money, power, prestige, a safety net. They're heroes. . . . But for a woman. What guy wants to put up with that shit? . . . I've told people before that I'm a bartender and I can have a great conversation with them. But once I tell them I'm a surgeon, forget it.

Like many of the other female residents I followed, Karen thought that she couldn't quite be an Iron Man no matter how hard she tried.

Despite the particular difficulties they faced, not all female residents supported the work-hours change. Some did their best to think and act like "one of the guys," despite the challenges involved. For example, several female residents tried to be Iron Men by going to male residents' bachelor parties at strip joints. These attempts inevitably backfired; in one case a male resident got drunk and, in his confusion, "grabbed the boobs of [a female resident] rather than the stripper."

MALE GENERAL SURGERY RESIDENTS

Other-specialty and female residents had reason to question traditional surgical roles, authority relations, and legitimating accounts given the marginal status assigned to them. Male general surgery residents who fell into three groups that I will call "Family Men," "Egalitarian Men," and "Patient-Centered Men" questioned these institutions for a different reason. They felt constrained from acting out social roles, other than that of Iron Man, that they valued.

Because the Iron Man's sense of self was so strongly shaped by the actions and understandings of the surgical community, Iron Men experienced little role conflict. Before the work-hours change, surgical residency was a total institution.[6] Residents went home only to sleep; often they did not leave the hospital for days on end. Their personal narratives—how they would tell others who they were—were closely bound to the narratives of the surgical community. Many of the male residents I followed had wives or significant others who took care of all the work at home—grocery shopping, cooking, cleaning, and childcare. The Iron Men who talked about these matters suffered from no apparent remorse or guilt because of this arrangement. The Iron Man wives I talked to, while they didn't like it, in general accepted it as a matter of course.

Some male residents, on the other hand, talked about the disparity between how they were expected to act in surgical residency and how they were expected to act in other domains of life. This disparity created tension. For example, as we sat in the otherwise empty surgical lounge one evening, a Family Man resident told me how "pathetic" it seemed to him that at the end-of-the year ceremony the week before, all the outgoing chiefs had seemed to be apologizing to their families. He went on to say about himself:

> I don't want to look back after seven years and think that I've abused anyone or kept asking for favors. I think it's totally unfair. And I'm not saying I've never done it, because I have. I'm much less inclined to send my parents gifts now on Mother's Day and Father's Day and on their birthdays than I was before residency. You're so busy and they understand that. But it's sort of an

abuse. . . . When it comes down to it, I still like believing that I can have a life outside of work. I don't want to do the same thing all the time every day and not have anything else. I want to have balance, whether it be kids or the opportunity to go play soccer with my friends.

Male residents with children found it particularly difficult to conform to the Iron Man ideal, however much they may have aspired to it. One male chief explained:

It's different for us than it was for these senior attendings. When we get home at night, our wives have been working, and they've gotten home earlier than us and started with the kids. And the minute you walk in the door, you're a dad. You're changing diapers or putting the kids to bed or doing their baths. And you're trying to help around the house. Then comes all of the other stuff you have to do, like reading, you're doing once everyone else has gone to bed. Working these hours means you end up asking a lot of favors.

Jeff Lucas, an incoming chief at Calhoun, said, "You want to get home to see your kids. You want to see your kids grow up. You have to learn this stuff to be a good surgeon, but you also don't want to be here doing worthless, ridiculous things that aren't, to me, part of my education. When I'm thirty-four years old and have three kids and am getting paid nothing to do it, then it's just not worth it. And I think that's something that people have to address now."

While Family Men supported change so they could better integrate their work and personal lives, Egalitarian Men simply did not feel comfortable with the macho Iron Man ideal. Ben Davis at Advent exemplified the views of the Egalitarian Men. One night I was sitting at dinner in the hospital cafeteria with him and his girlfriend, Alice, an obstetrics and gynecology resident. Alice described Ben as a very special person in the culture of general surgery. "Because he brings a certain levity to the situation. Usually you should have a straight face and be serious when you are in a room of general surgeons. He is the opposite. He likes to make the juniors feel comfortable."

Ben knew what he'd have to do to get the Iron Man rewards. The prescriptions for Iron Man behavior were clear. But he wasn't willing to act like an Iron Man to get these benefits. "When you get to be a higher level," he explained, "there's a certain personality you're expected to carry. Machismo becomes very important."

"What do you mean by machismo?" I asked. He replied:

You know, you never go home. Like, oh, your wife had a baby? And you're here two days afterwards. Or you're aggressive and yelling at people, intimidating people. You never call a consult. You want to always be in the OR. You want to do every case. Or you're talking all the time about the past. You know, like "We walked uphill both ways to school." Or "I was here when Bob McKenna was chief resident. His wife and family moved to Ohio ahead of him. And instead of finding a place to stay, he moved right into the call room." Macho, right? Some residents get away with not being good because they know how to act macho and are part of the "in group." . . . They're cruisers. And you're like "You're not even a good resident." But they can do well because they're in with the chiefs and the attendings. They can be more successful. . . . The chief will let them do some case when they're a second year that should be for a fourth year. Like they get to do a carotid [removal of plaque from an artery]. Or when it comes time to get a fellowship or a job, the attendings will pull for them. But I refuse to act that way.

There was a third group of male residents who did not feel comfortable with the traditional Iron Man persona: male residents who referred to themselves as "patient-centered." Like the Family Men who wanted more time with their girlfriends, wives, and children and the Egalitarian Men who were uncomfortable in the stereotypic macho role of Iron Men, these residents had difficulty maintaining a consistent personal narrative as they went about their daily work. Patient-Centered Men were genuinely interested in caring for patients one on one, and they enjoyed doing work up on the patient floors.

I did afternoon floorwork with one such resident at Bayshore, Kiran Mehta. Kiran's practices characterized those of the male residents who told me that they supported change because they were "patient-centered." Kiran said that he thought it was important to see patients at all different stages, pre-operatively, in the OR, on the floor, even after they went home. Some kinds of complications didn't show up until weeks later, he said, and he wanted to know about them.

As I followed him, I noted that he spent more time with each patient than did many of the other residents I had previously followed. Kiran took time to ask them how they felt, explain their procedures, and listen sympathetically to their complaints and concerns. He thought it was important to learn the essential information about every patient, not just enough to get by. He told me that he enjoyed taking care of the patients and liked going to clinic once a week to see them on their visits to the attendings—something that many residents hated because they wanted to be in the OR whenever possible.

As Kiran talked about why he liked face-to-face work with patients, he called the care coordinator who helped to place the patients in rehab centers or nursing homes. "Wafter is going home tomorrow with VNA services. I could send her today, but she is resistant. Johnson is going home today. Lyons is going to be with us for a few days. I'm putting in a PT consult for her. It might be worth doing a rehab screen for her." Among the Iron Men, the floorwork Kiran was doing was not "real work"—it was scutwork, tedious and dull. But for Kiran it was meaningful, even if it was not valued by his superiors and most of his colleagues. They valued being a hard worker, a skilled surgeon in the OR. Kiran sighed. "The seniors don't really know who works and who doesn't. So it ends up being all about whether you live for the OR. I don't."

A handful of other residents took Kiran's view as well, agreeing with him that focusing exclusively on being in the OR was done at the expense of resolving patient management issues. This view was expressed by another male resident on his way to afternoon rounds:

> I think managing patients on the floor is important. But it is not valued by general surgeons because it is considered the touchy-feely part of training. If you don't see someone's guts splayed open, if you don't take knife to skin, then it is not considered important. People think that unless you are doing an operation everything else is scut.
>
> The only thing I would call scutwork is if someone said "Go get me a cup of coffee." I don't think that anybody should be above tracking down a film, transferring a patient, looking up labs, drawing labs when they need to be drawn, doing transfer orders. People think that unless you are doing an operation, everything else is scutwork. . . . The nurses have told me that patients tell the attendings that they like me, but I never hear that from the attendings. They never say "Good job with that patient." They don't mention it.

Patient-centered residents also suggested that the individualistic surgical persona wasn't well suited to delivering care in today's environment. They noted that specialists are now plentiful and many different kinds of providers are involved in patient care. In this environment, they said, communication and learning to work effectively with other care providers rather than independent, authoritative decision making were essential. One patient-centered reformer noted:

> I've heard from day one that what distinguishes surgery is that surgeons can take care of anything. You'll hear people say, "He's not only the best surgeon I know, he's also the best internist I know." That's such bullshit. It's so demeaning to other doctors who are expert in something to think you can do it as well they can. It's just so wrong. Even here on the surgical service, every time things happen that are outside of the realm of surgery, [it's] "Yeah, you can take care of things." If somebody's having a heart attack, I'm not saying you can't do something about it. But if I were having a heart attack, would I want me to take care of myself? No. And if I had diabetes, would I want me to take care of my diabetes? No. I can do it, but I don't do it anywhere near as well. That's why we ask for expert consults from cardiology and endocrine every day on all these patients. To suggest that surgeons can do everything themselves is just ridiculous.

HIGH PERCENTAGE OF INTERNAL REFORMERS

I have described the surgical core and the periphery in the hospitals I studied. Before the night float programs were introduced in the three hospitals, I conducted face-to-face interviews with 81 percent of the residents who would be working under the new programs on the general surgery services.[7] I asked residents whether or not they supported a work-hours reduction in their hospital. I followed this question with another about how they thought reduced work hours would affect outcomes they thought important, outcomes such as patient care, education, and work-personal life integration.

As figure 4.1 shows, all the incoming interns I talked to at the three hospitals were supportive of reform. They felt that not only the quality of their own work life but also the quality of patient care and resident education would improve when they began working fewer hours. (The labels in the figure suggest each resident's primary concern, but of course in real life the categories are not mutually exclusive: a person could be both a new intern and an egalitarian male.)[8]

All the other-specialty residents I talked to were also supportive of reform. The primary reason they gave was that they thought the reduction

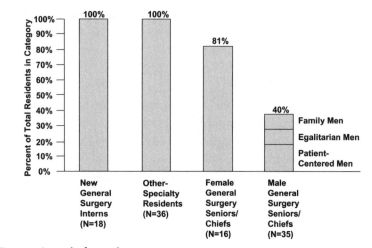

Figure 4.1. Internal reformers by category
N = number of residents interviewed at the three hospitals prior to the introduction of the night float programs.

in hours would lead general surgical residents to value other-specialty residents more highly. They also hoped that efficiency in floorwork (one of their strengths) would become more highly respected and that residents from their group would no longer be seen as inferior to general surgery residents since all of them now would be working eighty hours a week. Having more time for personal life was a secondary goal for them.

Most female general surgery chief and senior residents (81 percent across the three hospitals) were supportive of reform for the same fundamental reason: they hoped to improve their disadvantaged position in the surgical social world. They also wanted to have more time for their personal lives. One female resident noted: "In the new system, it will no longer be possible for people to get ahead by acting the most macho or living in the hospital. Instead, it will be about 'Are you efficient? Can you prioritize effectively?' . . . I think that this is going to be positive for women in surgery. . . . And I think that it will be good for everyone to be forced to add some more balance to their lives."

Finally, 40 percent of the male general surgery chief and senior residents at the three hospitals supported reform. Their primary goal varied depending on whether they were Patient-Centered Men (17 percent of male general surgery chiefs and seniors), Egalitarian Men (12 percent), or Family Men (11 percent).

It is striking that only the incoming interns supported work-hours re-form for the reasons that had motivated reform in the first place. While external reformers had won new regulation by framing current practices as unsafe for patients and harmful to residents, no internal reformers except for those in the intern subgroup said they supported work-hours reduction because it would improve patient safety or their own health or education.

Perhaps this should not be surprising. As trainees hoping to join the surgical profession, internal reformers who had been residents for more than a year had a vested interest in not admitting that the quality of patient care and of their own education had been impaired all along. Instead, they stressed quality of work and personal life as the problems that needed to be solved and asserted that while reducing resident work hours would not necessarily improve patient care or resident education, it would not harm them either. For example, one male reformer related:

> I think the changes are great and long overdue. . . . I think people's family lives go to ruin because of [the hours]. People's personal lives are nonex-istent. You don't have time to see anyone. It is ridiculous. . . . Any other person would think even eighty hours is crazy. . . . If we have good signouts we can make it work. Patient care won't be improved, but it will not be made worse. . . . Now we can go home and read about a case. We may see less since we won't be staying overnight. But over time, we will see enough. And we will be fresh. In some ways, we may learn more as a result. . . . It will also be great to be more awake when I'm outside the hospital. I am looking forward to it.

But this work-personal life integration frame was not as persuasive as the Iron Men's compelling patient care and education frames described in the last chapter. The lack of tailored frames supporting change was a problem that internal reformers would need to overcome.

Just as the frames that the external social movement had provided were not useful to internal reformers, so the reformer identities these external reformers had created were not helpful either. As noted in chapter 2, the identities of the overtired resident and the public advocate opposed to the medical establishment, while useful to external reformers, were not helpful to internal reformers.

Because the resources created by external reformers were not tailored for use by surgical residents inside teaching hospitals, they ended up not

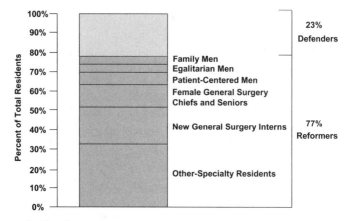

Figure 4.2. Residents by category
N = 105 residents interviewed at the three hospitals before the night float programs were introduced.

being very useful in allowing internal reformers in different subgroups at the three hospitals to see themselves as a collective group with similar reasons for wanting change.[9] The lack of tailored reformer frames and identity helps to explain why, when such a high percentage of residents at the three hospitals were internal reformers (77 percent across the three hospitals; see figure 4.2), the internal reformers initially blamed themselves rather than the system for their troubles and did not even begin to attempt change until it was officially mandated by directors.

Before the new programs were introduced, the beliefs of the internal reformers in each subgroups at the three hospitals were the same. Advent, Bayshore, and Calhoun had similar numbers of senior and chief resident reformers and similar numbers of interns who were beneficiaries of change.[10]

*   *   *

At the three hospitals, residents who held inferior positions in the surgical social world or who had other social identities that conflicted with the Iron Man role privately questioned the actions prescribed by traditional institutions. Internal reformers included incoming interns who did not yet understand traditional surgical principles, other-specialty residents for whom general surgery was not their ultimate career path, female residents, and male residents who wanted to take on personal responsibilities outside the hospital, who were uncomfortable with the macho Iron Man persona, or who saw themselves as patient-centered. There were high numbers of internal reformers at the three hospitals, but they did not act on their sense of a need for reform until their directors officially mandated change. As we will see in the next chapter, internal reformers *would* attempt change once directors mandated it. But Iron Men would not sit idly by as these insurgents challenged their treasured identity, trampled over their hard-won authority, and ran roughshod over their cherished beliefs.

PART TWO

COLLECTIVE COMBAT

5

Defending Stability

In the months leading up to the introduction of the night float program at the three hospitals, attendings and residents chose sides in the work-hours fight. But it wasn't until the directors launched the new program at the beginning of the resident year in July that the war began in earnest. Once the programs were introduced, internal reformers began to support change openly and Iron Men became active defenders of the status quo. The first victory at all three hospitals went to the defenders.

The night float programs were designed both to allow residents in all years to dramatically reduce the number of nights spent on call and to allow interns (who had historically worked the longest hours) to shorten their workdays so that all residents would be working eighty hours per week. Reducing the number of nights spent on call proved easy to do at all three hospitals, since the surgical directors had successfully negotiated with other departments to free up surgical residents to staff the night float programs. Substitution of one resident for another in the call schedule had been done frequently in the past, and this change was seen as merely a broader set of substitutions. Shortening intern workdays was much more difficult to accomplish.

The official rules of the night float program required new interns to hand off any uncompleted work to night floats and leave the hospital at 6 p.m. Perhaps not surprisingly, at all three hospitals defenders of the status quo assigned to the night float position resisted intern handoffs. As subordinates in a rigidly hierarchical system, interns obeyed these superiors and ceased attempting handoffs when interacting with them.

However, reformer night floats encouraged intern handoffs. So we might have expected that interns would learn to gauge the stance of their night float interaction partners and act accordingly. Instead, by about a month after program introduction, interns at all three hospitals had ceased attempting to hand off work altogether. Why?

The interns' actions were shaped by their alignment with professional rather than organizational goals. As newcomers accountable to multiple levels of supervisors and different supervisors with each rotation, the new interns wanted to impress not only the night float member on their current general surgery service but also the attending, chief, and senior resident on their current service and those on services they would be assigned to in the future. As new recruits to the surgical profession, interns wanted to learn not only about their hospitals' rules but also about their profession's standards for appropriate and inappropriate conduct. And as professional trainees, interns cared about not only improving their quality of work life but also gaining access to training and social acceptance by others in their professional group.[1]

In this chapter I will explain how defenders at the three hospitals capitalized on the new interns' concerns about professional reputations, roles, and rewards to dissuade them, at least initially, from attempting to use the night float programs that had been designed to benefit them. The 23 percent of residents who were defenders were bolstered by virtually all the attendings. Attendings and defender residents protected the status quo using four tactics: preempting program use, preventing program use, punishing program use, and organizing with one another.

PREEMPTING PROGRAM USE

During new intern orientation week at the end of June, the directors at Advent, Bayshore, and Calhoun introduced the night float programs in "grand rounds" meetings of all surgical attendings and residents.[2] Because it was the incoming chiefs who would need to manage the work on their services in new ways, directors assigned them responsibility for program implementation. Directors made it clear that the night float programs were designed to reduce residents' work hours and that night floats were responsible for all work on the general surgery services from 6 p.m. to 6 a.m. nightly. Reformer night floats embraced the program, encouraging interns to hand off by referencing the new rules and telling interns that it was the night floats' job to cover all routine work starting at 6 p.m.

But the new interns were concerned about their developing reputations more than about how their current night float team member expected them to behave. In this environment, defenders effectively preempted interns' use of the night float program by outlining their expectations for how interns should act. They also gossiped about interns who dared to hand off work—thus warning others about what would happen to their reputations if they failed to live up to expectations. On one of the first days of the new residency year, I saw a dramatic example of this expectation-setting. It was a little before 4 in the afternoon, and the new interns were packed into a basement room waiting for a talk by Iron Man attending Jack McLaughlin. At exactly 4 pm, Jack strode in wearing green scrubs and a surgical cap, a long white coat, and a surgical face mask down around his neck. He immediately began to fire off rules for the new residents. In doing so, he preemptively instructed the interns not to call traditional long hours practices unfair, not to blame night floats if they did not complete routine work overnight (even though, of course, the purpose of the new system was to create a team that would complete these routine tasks), and not to claim their new rights of reduced hours. In short, he implicitly told them not to use the night float program if they wanted to build their reputations as good interns: "I'm Dr. McLaughlin, one of the general surgery attendings. I'm available twenty-four hours a day, seven days a week. My pager is on twenty-four hours a day. If you have a problem, call me or page me. I want to know about it. The last thing we want is an unhappy intern."

Jack's kind words about his open-door policy were completely contradicted by his posture and tone of voice—and by what came next. He was a tightly wound ball of intensity as he barked out his standards and views:

> Be organized. Keep yourself organized. When your chief asks you a question, you don't want to be shuffling through your pockets or looking down at your scrub pants for an answer. There are two kinds of interns: those who write things down and those who forget. Always have a pen, and write everything your chief says down. The intern is the workhorse of the team. You need to work harder than everyone else, be available longer than anyone else.
>
> Be prompt. When rounds are at 6 a.m. don't show up at 6:05. If you've always been late your whole life, set your clock ahead. We run on a tight

schedule, and if the chief has set one and a half hours for rounds, he needs every minute. Don't show up at 6 with only half of your patients' numbers. Get here at whatever hour you need to in order to be ready. Also in the OR— nothing ticks an attending off more than having to drape and prep his own patient. If you aren't there to do it, some attendings will tell you to go, you've lost that procedure.

Be humble and respectful. Over the next six months, you'll make your reputation at Advent. The last thing you want to do in your first week is piss off some OR nurse who has been here for twenty years. If you do, she'll be operating with Goodwin [the surgery department director] and tell him what you did. He'll call me and say "What's the story with so-and-so? I hear he's a jerk." And next time Goodwin is at a function and reads your name tag, that's the first thing he is going to think about. . . . You don't know who is important and who isn't at first. So be careful and be humble. Be pleasant, be courteous. You don't want to start a seven-year relationship the wrong way. The difference between four hours of sleep and zero hours of sleep is your relationship with the nurses. If you are disrespectful, you'll be called all night about a normal potassium, a normal urine output, a normal blood pressure. Word gets around, and if you piss off one person, everyone will know.

Trust no one; expect nothing. You are responsible for your patients. . . . If Bill tells you to go home and he will take care of things, don't show up the next morning and find out that one of Goodwin's patients hasn't been pre-opped. The chief should never hear from an intern that "Oh, it's someone else's fault. The nurse didn't get the data," or "The consult service didn't show up." You are responsible for the nurse getting the data. You are responsible for the consult service showing up. You may need to page Neuro five times in order to get them there, but you need to get them there before rounds in the afternoon. You are responsible for your patients twenty-four hours a day. You own that patient. There are two acceptable answers to any question: either "Yes, I've done it" or "No, I didn't do it and I'll do it right away."

Be in perpetual motion. Don't say, "I'll have time between cases to check numbers, so I'm going to go for a cappuccino, watch TV, take a nap." Inevitably, something will blow up and you won't have time to get things before rounds. Check your labs and studies before doing anything else. You'll be inefficient in the beginning, and you need to do things right away in order to get them done.

We are excited to have you. You're here because you wanted to be here. We have that luxury. We are not like some middle-tier programs that are scrambling to fill slots with people who would rather be elsewhere. The first days will be scary, and there will be some reworking. You have the team supporting you.

Work hard. Bring us praise. Good habits start day one and bad habits are hard to break. Work hard. Put your nose to the grindstone, and you'll do well here. See you on Wednesday night at the Steakhouse. We'll throw back a few cold ones and celebrate your last week of freedom.

Here, even before the interns donned their scrubs for the first time, Jack had indoctrinated them into the traditional surgical intern identity of workhorse that justified exceptionally long work hours. He recast any future complaints they might make as resulting from personality clashes with nurses or their own inefficiencies, not from lack of compliance with the new work-hours regulations. And he threatened them with retaliation: if they tried to act in new ways, teaching would be withheld from them or they would have to face the wrath of the surgery department director.[3] In doing so, he hoped to preempt intern attempts to use the new night float program.

Defender chiefs set similar expectations during morning and afternoon rounds when a new intern rotated onto their service for the first time. For example, at Bayshore during her first rotation, Linda got some tips from her chief about how to be most effective. "By morning rounds at 6 a.m. you should have your notes written. Notes are the bane of our existence. In the morning, put in orders and labs. By noon, run around and see the patients and go to the OR, do a few things. Do it fast."

By telling Linda to do her notes before morning rounds, Mark was implicitly telling her to come in at 4 a.m. to pre-round (check on patients before morning rounds began at 6 a.m.) even though the rules of the new system required that night floats do the pre-rounding. By telling her to be fast, he was implicitly telling her that if she had not finished all her routine work by 6 p.m. when she was due to sign out, it was her own fault for not being more efficient.

Defenders also discouraged handoffs to night float members by gossiping to interns about other interns who had attempted them. One night I followed defender night float Tom Wilson at Advent. He was covering two services, and the intern on the first service had handed off several pre-ops for him to do. The intern on the second service, Margaret, paged him to sign out at 7:30 p.m. She had stayed late to finish all of the pre-ops on her service rather than handing them off to Tom.

TOM: Nice work getting all of your patients tucked away—unlike my other
    intern, who signed out to me an hour and a half ago.
MARGARET: [incredulous] You're kidding?
TOM: Oh, yeah. Unbelievable.

As a means of social control, Tom's gossip, with its implicit threat of
sanction from powerful community members, was an especially effective
preemption tactic given the small, stable, and outwardly homogenous character of the surgical occupational community. In the fishbowl of Advent,
Margaret knew who the other intern was even though Tom did not name
her. Knowing that they could be gossiped about, that their reputations could
be sullied, was enough to make interns think twice before making handoff
attempts.

PREVENTING PROGRAM USE

Defenders also resisted change by actually refusing to accept handoffs when
interns attempted them. While the tactic of preempting program use was
used by attendings, defender chiefs, and defender senior residents, the
tactic of preventing program use was available only to the defender senior
residents who were serving on the night float team. The official rules of the
night float program required interns to hand off whatever work was not
completed by 6 p.m. to the night float covering their service, and the same
rules required night floats to accept handoffs of any and all work that had
not been completed.

But as new recruits to the surgical profession, interns cared less about
official rules and more about demonstrating appropriate conduct for their
surgical role and their position in relation to other professionals. Defenders
capitalized on the interns' professional aspirations to prevent program use.
They used traditional surgical legitimating accounts to label long-standing
practices fair. They drew on traditional surgical roles to deflect blame for
their failure to support the new program. And they invoked traditional
surgical authority relations to discourage intern claims for change. For example, when an intern tried to hand off post-ops to a defender night float,
the night float cited "continuity of care" in explaining to the intern why it
was inappropriate to do so: "In surgery, things can turn on a dime. . . . If
you're a patient's doctor, you need to know them inside and out. That patient's care depends on you knowing every detail. The problem with handoffs is that things fall through the cracks."

Similarly, defender night floats argued that resident education would suffer under the new handoff rules. One Calhoun night float told interns that they weren't factory workers who could punch a clock and leave work. If they handed off their patients, he insisted, they would never learn to take responsibility for them. "You need to learn, 'I'm a doctor. I will stay until the work gets done, until the patient is OK, and if they are not OK, I'm not going leave, even if it's a hundred hours in a row.'"

Defenders used other tactics. They justified their refusal to accept hand-offs on the grounds that handoffs violated traditional roles in surgery. They labeled routine work—post-ops (checking patients several hours after they came out of the OR to make sure they were recovering well from surgery), pre-ops (checking paperwork on patients scheduled to go to the OR the next day and ordering any necessary additional tests), admits (admitting new patients to the hospital), and pre-rounding (gathering patient data in the morning before rounds)—"intern work" and argued that it was fair for interns to stay until 9 or 10 at night and arrive at 4 the next morning be-cause they needed to "pay their dues" just as the chiefs and seniors had done before them.

For example, one night at 8, Steve Everett, a defender night float cover-ing the vascular surgery service at Bayshore, was paged by a nurse about admitting a newly arrived patient. The nurse had first paged the intern on the service who was still in the hospital taking care of pre-ops for the next day. But since it was past 6 p.m., the intern had told her to page the night float instead. Steve was furious. He told me that admits were "intern work" and the intern should have taken the nurse's call and put in the admit or-ders himself. Steve paged the intern. "Listen, there was a patient admitted to Michelli [an attending]. Don't buck everything to me. I already did my internship, and I don't need to do it again." Steve hung up and said to me, "Even now, he is giving me attitude."

When I asked defender night floats about their actions, they intimated that they felt that routine work like this was inappropriate for members of their standing in the residency organization. And they drew on tradi-tional ideas about education to justify their actions. One explained: "They shouldn't be expecting me to do this stuff for them. I did my internship three years ago. I don't need to do it again. There's not the pride of ownership that there was before, where you couldn't go home until the work was done. The problem with this signout business is they don't learn to be efficient. I could do these things, but it takes away from their education."

In addition to naming the traditional signout practice fair and deflecting blame for rejecting handoffs, defender night floats drew on the traditional hierarchy of seniors over juniors to discourage handoff attempts. They arrived at the hospital long past 6 p.m., minimizing contact with interns. They "ran the list" (reviewed the list of patients and associated surgical conditions) as rapidly as possible to signal that they wanted to hear about potential emergencies only and not about routine tasks that needed to be done. They rolled their eyes when an intern tried to hand off the checking of tests or films.

Anand Roy, a defender night float at Advent, was a master at drawing on traditional authority relations to discourage handoff attempts. One night as I was following him, he rejected handoffs from interns on both of the services he was covering. He had arrived at the hospital shortly after 6p.m., but rather than paging the interns to ask for their signout, he'd gone to the surgical lounge to hang out with another night float. They had talked about the Victoria's Secret underwear show that would be on TV later that evening and what terrible surgeons the new interns were going to be since they were no longer on call every third night. At 8:15 p.m., more than two hours after she should have left the hospital, Maya, the other-specialty intern on the GI surgery service, tracked him down. During signout, she asked him to get films for one of the operations that would occur the next day on the service, and he refused. According to Anand, getting films was "intern work."

MAYA: These films need to be printed.

ANAND: [rolls his eyes] What for?

MAYA: For the OR. He [the attending] has been wanting them. So if they have a film, you print them.

ANAND: [implicitly rejecting the handoff attempt] I always think that's a waste.

Soon after, Nick, the intern from the other service Anand was covering, came by to sign out. During signout, Nick asked Anand to call for a test. Anand rejected this handoff attempt as well:

NICK: The only thing to sign out is to call and ask if it is possible to do a Doppler [ultrasound] tonight.

ANAND: You know they won't do it.

NICK: Josh [the chief] wanted to call.

ANAND: [implicitly refusing] I'll page him for you right now.

NICK: We just need an incomplete study, only one leg.

ANAND: [drawls to show displeasure] Allllright. You can make your case, but they won't do it.

NICK: Really?

ANAND: Dipshit [referring to the reformer chief]. That's an example of flogging the system. It is unnecessary. It is 8:30 [p.m.]. It's not good for the patient, not good for anybody, and it can wait until tomorrow.

Anand dialed and handed the phone to Nick. He talked to the other night float in the lounge while Nick requested the study. Nick hung up.

ANAND: What did they say?

NICK: They are going to do it.

ANAND: [incredulous] They are? Both legs?

NICK: No, Josh just wanted one.

ANAND: Wow, I'm impressed.

Nick then tried to hand off his cards to Anand so that Anand would update them overnight. Even handing off the notecards was frowned upon:

ANAND: I don't need those cards. What am I going to do, read those cards if someone is coding [dying]?

NICK: No, to check meds or something.

ANAND: It only helps you if you write them. I know that Ben [reformer night float] and those guys treat them like the Bible and carry them everywhere. I don't need them.

By refusing to get films, call for tests, or take patient cards, Anand prevented Maya and Nick from using the night float program as mandated by the official rules. And by rolling his eyes, he made them feel uncomfortable and out of line for even having attempted a handoff.

One may wonder whether defender night floats blatantly ignored the formal rules in this way when interacting in public spaces. They did. Defender night floats were quite open about their refusal to take handoffs in front of defenders and reformer residents alike. It is likely that night floats would not have ignored the official rules had a director been present, but I never saw a director present during a signout interaction; signouts occurred in the resident domains of the surgical resident lounge and less busy corners of the patient floors. Night floats felt comfortable rejecting handoffs in front of reformer residents because attendings and most chief residents supported resistance and because traditional surgical accounts justified their resistance.

Why didn't the directors in the three hospitals intervene when it became clear that the interns were not using the night float program to change their signout practices? They did not get involved because they did not know that the program was not being used by the residents as intended. At this point even reformer chiefs did not tell the directors that the system was being flouted; they explained to the directors that they were "still working out the logistics."[4]

And why didn't reformer chiefs alert directors that interns were not handing off to seniors? They did not do so because they had not yet developed new frames, a new identity, and a sense of efficacy that supported handoffs. At this point, reformer chiefs themselves were unsure whether it was possible to hand off without undermining patient care and resident education. And too, telling the directors that the program was not being followed conflicted with the traditional surgical resident identity. In the surgical culture, talking to directors about problems on one's team indicated that a chief did not "have his house in order."

PUNISHING PROGRAM USE

In addition to preventing program use, defenders resisted change by punishing interns who attempted handoffs. External reformers who had pressed for new regulation had argued that it would improve residents' quality of work life because they would get to work fewer hours. But as professional trainees, interns cared not only about improving the quality of their work life but also about being accepted by their professional group and gaining access to valued training opportunities.

Attendings, defender chiefs, and defender seniors exploited these desires by punishing interns who used the night float programs; they shamed them in front of their peers and withheld social affiliation and teaching. One Bayshore intern related how one of the night float members lost his temper and shamed her in front of other residents when she tried to hand off work: "Scott got mad and told me that was ridiculous. We were up on the fifth floor, and he did it in front of a bunch of other residents."

When defender chiefs heard from defender night floats that interns on their teams had tried to sign out routine work, they loudly and publicly drew attention to them through what they called "beatings." One defender explained: "You do the screaming for the effect with others rather than for that individual. You want to draw attention to the fact that 'Moron is over here.' Now, if I'm with a resident one on one, there's no point in me elevating my voice and being like 'Moron's over here.' Then, it's more like 'Listen you knucklehead, you're really fucking up, and you need to get your shit together because I'm not going to tolerate this anymore.'"

Defenders also withheld social affiliation from interns who attempted handoffs. At Advent, intern Stephanie Lewis was punished by defender chiefs and seniors when she attempted to hand off to the night float the work she had not accomplished by 6 p.m. Stephanie was an other-specialty resident spending a year training in general surgery before moving on to urology. Defenders punished her by withholding social affiliation. They excluded her in a variety of ways: not paging her to ask her to lunch, not inviting her to their parties, communicating with her only about work tasks. By stigmatizing Stephanie, defenders set an example for other interns, who often chose not to pollute themselves by socializing with a social outcast. In this way, they not only punished interns who attempted change but also highlighted behavior that was outside the bounds of acceptability for the group.

In addition, defenders withheld training opportunities, punishing uncooperative interns by not assigning them interesting cases. Advent defender chief Matt Baker explained to me why he didn't assign the best cases to Stephanie: "A lot of it is who the chiefs like. Who do I want to hook up? People want to operate. When I throw the juniors a bone, it is because they have worked hard for me. Like Peter. I let him do a splenectomy last week. That was a total bone. It is a third- or fourth-year case." Attendings at the three hospitals decreased the amount of time they spent teaching interns whose reputations had been sullied. Concerning one intern who had fallen out of favor, an attending at Calhoun confessed, "I could have spent an extra ten or fifteen minutes doing a case with him, giving him a little more time, making it a better experience for him, but I didn't do it."

Someone not familiar with the strong hierarchy in surgery (and the attractive awards awaiting those who survived surgical residency) might be surprised that interns at the three hospitals did not rebut the claims made by attendings and defender chiefs and seniors. One could imagine interns making countercharges such as "If long hours are required, why are you leaving?" "If doctors need to take responsibility for their patients, why don't you need to order the tests required for good patient care?" Or, more mildly, "The new rules require that I hand off any work not completed at 6:00 p.m." Yet as law and society scholars have shown, strong hierarchies with a hands-off approach at the top and long-standing cultural practices such as shaming make it easy for middle managers to resist change. Authoritative commands typically flow down the hierarchy but not up, and when subordinates face difficulties with their superiors, they most often react by either doing nothing or by engaging in covert action.[5] Indeed, as we will see in the next chapter, interns and other internal reformers often rebutted defender claims when interacting in private spaces with others whom they knew were sympathetic to change.

ORGANIZING WITH OTHER DEFENDERS

Even though directors were not actively confronting those resisting the new program, attendings, defender chiefs, and defender seniors were taking some career risks by disobeying the new rules since directors at the three hospitals were pressing for change. Defenders needed to persuade one another to take such risks on behalf of the group as a whole, and they needed to craft a set of tactics they could use to resist systematically in any number of situations. Defenders built commitment to the defender group in part by adopting the identity provided by the external countermovement that had fought against the patients' rights and residents' rights groups. As described in the introduction, the external countermovement, led by those within the surgical profession, had developed a public identity of responsible surgeons who were committed to protecting patients; they contrasted themselves to outsiders who did not understand the needs of patients and residents. Calhoun defender chief Tahir Azim explained that those opposed to the new regime were called "old school" because of their belief in the tradition that interns should stay in the hospital as long as it took to get the job done. Defenders inside the three hospitals used the "old school" identity to build a unified group with one another.

Defenders also built commitment by creating feelings of belonging to a collective that had high status, a status that was deserved because it was achieved by living up to standards that were higher, more honorable, and more efficacious than the standards of those who sought change. This was a powerful identity. Defenders portrayed themselves as the true "we," the Iron Men—that venerated and prestigious identity that historically had been so valued by the profession—and thus worthy of sitting atop the surgical society. The reformers they portrayed as a "they" who wanted to work fewer hours, work less hard, and learn less and who therefore deserved lower-status careers.

One of the defenders' tactics was to equate the reformers with "med-dies," medical residents (such as those training to be primary care physi-cians). Unlike surgical residency programs, medical residency programs traditionally had been structured around shorter hours and, hence, more handoffs. Defenders suggested that because of these handoffs, medical resi-dents were not as knowledgeable about their patients as surgical residents were. If work hours were reduced in surgery, surgical residents would be-come "just as bad" as medical residents. To surgical residents defending the status quo, it followed that if medical residents did not work as many hours as surgical residents, they clearly were not as well trained. The implica-tion was obvious. If the reformers succeeded in reducing hours, surgical residents would no longer be trained to "outthink and outperform" those in medical disciplines. They would all fall from grace.

As defenders drew distinctions between "us" and "them," they argued that their high status in the medical world was dependent on their willing-ness to work long hours to acquire the skills they would need to become good surgeons. One attending said: "We are the future leaders of American surgery. It's like being an astronaut. Only the best, the toughest, the bright-est get to go into space. And you feel like only the best, the brightest, the toughest, can train here. Because if it were easy, *everyone* would do it."

A third way defenders built commitment to the defender group was to tell stories to one another about how other care providers—anesthesiolo-gists and nurses, for instance—"lost it" while surgeons and surgical resi-dents remained calm and in control because they had learned surgery by working long hours. One attending told this story in front of an audience of several interns and senior residents. During his year as a chief, he had been called one night to the OR:

> I was the chief on Larkin [the trauma service] in house, sleeping up in the bunk, and Galiardo was the chief on Hughes [the GI surgery service]. Jones [an attending] was doing an emergency thyroid for some reason, and the patient arrested on the table. So Jones turned to the circulator [circulat-ing nurse] and said, "Dial 5-6326, tell Phillips to get his ass down here." The phone rings: "Yeah it's Room 12. Jones needs you down here." So I get down there. I go into the room; it was totally surreal. The anesthesia resident was crying in the corner. The anesthesia attending was staring at the monitor. Jones was barking out orders, doing chest compressions. And Galiardo was trying to put a line in the guy's spine. So I get in there, and the two of us re-suscitate the person and bring 'im back.

And it's just those types of things where, when all hope is lost, call the surgeon. Because you've been here seven years, you've done every other night, you've seen everything. You feel like you could keep a rock alive, because you've seen it all. And it's painful to get to that point where you feel that way, but you sort of feel like no one else can do as good a job as you. And it's not beating your chest, [taunts] "I'm better than you are." It's just, someone is coding, all right, well, open the chest. [He pantomimes being an incredulous onlooker.] "Oh my god." Well, yeah, we're going to do everything we can within our power to bring this person back. We're not going to leave any stone unturned.

The reason you can do it is that you've always been given that responsibility. Been given that much volume. Been pushed to the limit all the time. You know there comes a point where the fear is gone, where you lose that fear. It's an intensity thing. The intensity tells you how to triage stuff in your mind, tells you how to handle things, tells you how to manage things in an appropriate manner. It's like this patient needs a chest tube *now*. And boom, you pop a chest tube in in thirty seconds. This patient has a hole in their heart. No one else can get into the chest cavity. You can.

Telling this story of the glory days when surgical residents who had been trained in 120-hour workweeks handled emergencies effortlessly while doctors who had worked fewer hours cowered in a corner, the attending painted an attractive picture of "we" who were "cool under pressure," had "nerves of steel," and were "unflappable" in the face of high-stakes situations because of long work hours during training.

The creation of a collective identity led defenders to take personal risks on behalf of the group as a whole. But to block the change effectively, defenders also needed to develop common responses to attempts to use the night float program. What challenges would they accept and which would they ignore? Would they accept handoffs of some tasks but not others? Were there extenuating circumstances under which some might accept a handoff? What justifications would they develop and articulate for resisting these attempts?

While they did not formally plan out what responses to use and not to use, defenders did end up collectively strategizing and coordinating their resistance efforts during casual dinners in the cafeteria, discussions in the surgical lounge, hallway conversations, and other occasions on which they gathered. Night floats were not busy. They spent some of their downtime telling stories about their outrage at handoff attempts and sharing their own signout "policies" with one another. When I asked if they got together to discuss the change, one defender chief at Calhoun responded: "We'll sort of congregate down in the cafeteria. You sit down and talk and people tell stories and stuff like that. Basically we just blow off steam. So when the interns started trying get out of here at 5:59, of course we talked about it. . . . We needed to beat it into these guys that it wasn't acceptable."

I observed this sharing of tactics in action one August evening at Advent. Anand (third year), Tom (second year), and Samir (fourth year) on night float were having dinner in the cafeteria with Jill, a surgical resident on an ICU rotation. Anand said, "Radan [an intern] tried to hand off to me. So I told her, 'I won't do admits that came in before 4 [p.m.].' Anything before 4, they gotta do it." Tom chimed in, "My policy is they can't sign out to me until after rounds. I told them I refuse to get pages on patients I don't know anything about." By not taking admits and other scutwork that came in before 4 p.m. and not allowing interns to sign out until after rounds, night floats pressed interns to stay past 6 p.m. Interns in the OR could not begin floorwork until after they were out of the OR, and they often had a long list of tasks to do once they got out. Rounds were often held by defender chiefs after 6 p.m.

In these informal encounters, defenders also tried out possible justifications for resistance with one another. One night, as Felipe, a defender night float, was waiting for the fourth-floor elevator, Pam, another defender night float member, came out of the opposite elevator. They began talking about the interns. "I'm concerned about their work ethic," Felipe said. "They need to learn that these are their patients. Rather than at 4 [p.m.] they got an admit [new patient who needed to be admitted] but they know there is a night float coming on so they save it for the night float. When we were interns, we learned to be efficient and get it done."

Pam agreed. "I have a problem doing an admission if a patient got here at 3 [p.m.] and the interns are going home. They have it so much easier even when they work late. I'd rather sleep in my own bed for three hours than sleep ten hours here. I'm not going to do their pre-ops for them while they get out of here at 7 [p.m.]."

Felipe added, "They need to suck it up and be the workhorse. This new system is not forcing them to be responsible. When we were interns, you were responsible for the patient, and if the patient didn't do well you had to face the team, the attending, and the patient, and say, 'I didn't measure up.' They are not facing the responsibility they'll have as a chief or attending."

In addition to sharing tactics among themselves, the night float members worked to get defender chiefs to support these tactics by telling them stories to show that interns were "not taking responsibility for their patients" and were trying to hand off "intern work" to night float members. One night at Bayshore, I was following Scott, a defender night float, when Jim, a chief, came by. Scott told Jim that Woodson (the attending) had made another "stealth admit" (unexpected admission late in the day) and that Walker (the intern) had tried to hand off the admission to Scott. Scott complained that the new interns had attitudes and were arrogant. "I've got an intern who likes to buck all of his patients to me. It pisses off the nurses. And it's irritating. The nurses call me and I say, 'Call the intern,' and they say, 'I already did.'"

At Advent I observed the same strategy of defender night float members enlisting the help of defender chiefs. In early July, night float Daniel Cohen stopped chief Paul Robertson in the hall on his way out and complained, "It's a waste of time for night floats to come to rounds when they could be getting started on work." In fact, defender night floats often did not even arrive in the hospital until after 6 p.m., and as noted earlier, once they did arrive, they avoided signouts with interns until an hour or two later. They checked their e-mail and talked with one another while delaying intern signout.

AT THE END OF THE FIRST ROUND OF SKIRMISHES

By using these resistance tactics, defenders at the three hospitals were, at least initially, successful in pressuring each reformer into one of three categories. They converted some interns to defenders by teaching them what they considered appropriate behavior for surgical professionals in the intern position. Other reformers were silenced and hence prevented from attempting or supporting handoffs. A third group, only a handful in each hospital at this point, refused to be silenced, so defenders stigmatized them.

In the face of defender tactics, many interns simply stopped trying to use the night float programs. When they first had entered as residents, they had been ignorant of traditional surgical ideals. Defenders taught them about the problems associated with disobeying professional rules, and converts swiftly came to support traditional practices—in short, they came to believe that traditional ways of working produced the best patient care and the best resident education. "I try not to sign out much," one convert said. "It is hard to let someone else take care of your patients. It requires a good signout. People always make mistakes. So I'll stay until I feel like I've checked everything I need to." Another convert, who admired a defender chief, re-marked, "I think whatever they did with him, I want to experience the same thing so I can end up like him. I didn't come into surgical residency to make my life easier. I came here to learn. And whatever it takes to do that, that's what I'm gonna do."

Once the traditional practices, frames, and identity were internalized by converts as elements of their routine repertoire, they served as inner controls. External controls in the form of defender retaliations became un-necessary. Traditional practices were seen as fair. "The system" rather than individuals were to blame for long work hours, and "the system" came to be seen as both just and good.

The second subgroup of reformers—whom I will call secret reform-ers—also stopped attempting to use or support the night float program. Unlike converts, secret reformers stopped because they feared retribution from their superiors, who controlled access to their training and career placement. Interns who became secret reformers were no longer new to the hospitals and now understood the rules of the surgical social system. But they supported reform anyway for the same reasons that their more se-nior counterparts had from the beginning; secret reformer interns tended to be other-specialty residents, female general surgery residents, or male general surgery residents who were patient centered, egalitarian, or fam-ily men.

Secret reformer interns stopped overtly attempting change at this point in the year to avoid negative sanctions. One intern who initially had at-tempted handoffs said he had stopped trying because "reputation is impor-tant here. There is a lot of talking, and this is a small program. A lot of people don't say things to your face, but if you hand off then they tell others that this guy is weak." Overhearing these remarks, another intern agreed: "I don't hand off my work to others and go home because of pride and reputa-tion. If people trust you, they let you do more. And they look out for you." These sanction-oriented secret reformers strove to comply with traditional expectations:

> Being considered a good intern has nothing to do with what you know or how well you manage your patients. It is totally based on working hard and not handing stuff off. It's your attitude, not your ability. Like never passing off pre-ops to people. . . . This is where I live. I only go home to sleep. It sounds sick, but these people are like my family. The worst thing would be to not be respected by these guys.

In a system where residents' education depended on their winning the trust, guidance, and teaching of senior residents, chiefs, and attendings, secret reformer interns at the three hospitals chose not to hand off their work, and secret reformer seniors chose not to overtly support the night float program. One secret reformer senior told me that he was always trying to prove his competence to the "old-school people." If you could prove yourself, he said, then others would give you more latitude as well as support your promotions through fellowship recommendation letters. "First impressions matter," this resident said, "but so do last impressions. You're always trying to keep up the reputation you've built."

Finally, at the three hospitals at this point in the year, there was a small group—very small, three to five at most at each hospital—who could be classified as "overt reformers." These were reformer chiefs who did not care whether they were accepted by defenders and who were already expecting to leave their respective hospitals at the end of the year. By going public with their preferences, they still risked a good deal, as I have suggested. These overt reformers considered defender retaliations a threat, to be sure, but they continued to push for change. Why and how they did it is what I take up in the following chapter.

*   *   *

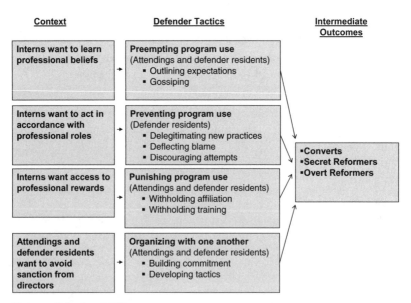

Figure 5.1. Defending stability

Defenders of the status quo at the three hospitals were attending chief and senior Iron Men who resisted change using a wide range of tactics; they took preemptive action so that many interns did not even attempt to use the night float programs, prevented handoffs when interns did attempt them, punished interns who did so, and coordinated with and supported other defenders (see figure 5.1). Given the defenders' coordinated and adamant resistance and their superior positions in the strict surgical hierarchy, it is not surprising that interns at the three hospitals stopped attempting hand-offs when in the presence of Iron Men. In fact, once we understand the importance of interns' alignment with professional rather than organizational goals, it is not even surprising that they would try to protect their professional reputations by stopping handoff attempts altogether, even in interactions with reformers. What remains puzzling is that some time after reformers at all three hospitals appeared to have been decisively defeated, reformers at Advent and Calhoun (but not Bayshore) began to act collectively for change. The next chapter explains how we can account for this turnaround.

6

Relationally
Mobilizing for
Change

Sanil Gupta, an intern at Advent, smiled as he headed toward the fourth-floor conference room for 5 p.m. rounds. Many of the chiefs didn't round until later, but his chief made a point of rounding early so the team members could finish up as much of their work as possible by 6 p.m.

When Sanil arrived, Carl Johnson, the senior resident on the vascular surgery service, was already there sitting at the computer. The conference room contained a wooden rectangular table and a small desk on which the computer sat. Deepak Patel, the chief, came in soon after, and Sanil started going down the list of patients, telling Deepak what had been done. "Taylor: afebrile, vital signs stable. Needs labs." Next patient. "Smith: Need to page Dr. Whetten about her to make sure we can send her home."

At all three hospitals, residents on each service gathered together every evening for "afternoon rounds" to review the post-operative patient care that had been carried out that day by the intern. Deepak's manner was consultative as they went down the list. After each patient, he asked, "So what do you want to do?" They would discuss each patient for a moment and move on. Sanil recorded the orders for each patient. Just as he finished going through his list, he was paged. A patient had arrived and needed to be admitted. He groaned inwardly. This was one of the worst pages for an intern. It meant your next hour had just gone out the door. You had to put your other duties on hold and deal with the arrival of this new, unexpected work. The residents called these arrivals "scuds" because they arrived like Scud missiles, coming out of nowhere and wreaking havoc.

Deepak said, "OK. You go. We can put the orders in and send that text page [text entered into computer and sent to a doctor or nurse]." Sanil hesitated, then ignored Deepak's offer for help and started typing the text page. This was intern work. But Deepak said, "Go, go." Sanil looked up but then started typing it in again. Deepak insisted, "Go. We'll take care of it." Sanil said, "OK," hesitated a moment more, then left to deal with the new patient. Since Carl was sitting at the computer, Deepak dictated the text page and Carl typed it in: "Smith's scan shows graft is wide open, going to send her home. Call if ?s [call if you have questions]. Thanks."

As Sanil headed up to the sixth floor to admit the new patient, he wondered whether he should have stayed to finish the orders. No, he decided, Deepak had been insistent about having Sanil leave the meeting to do the admit. Sanil needed to get used to this new kind of team. None of his previous chiefs would have offered to send a text page for an intern. Deepak often acted in this fashion. If he was down in radiology, he got films, and he sometimes did patient discharges, even though both of these tasks had traditionally been done only by interns. Deepak did so because he was trying to meet the demands of the new work-hours regulation. Carl, the senior on the service, also tried to do what was necessary to help everyone on the team finish their work by 6 p.m.

Sanil had rotated onto the vascular surgery service just four days earlier. His service was what I will call a "reformer-only service." Sanil didn't use this phrase, but he did notice that all of his new teammates were supportive of the work-hours regulation. Deepak and Carl supported the new regulation, and Sarah, the senior resident assigned to night float that month, supported it too.

Sanil told me he liked the fact that he was now leaving the hospital shortly after 6 p.m. and arriving shortly before 6 a.m., as the night float program rules specified. But he still wasn't used to how his new team worked with one another. Like Deepak, Carl did things that that were unusual for senior residents. He often helped out with routine tasks during the day, such as doing pre-ops and post-ops, or writing out discharge orders or consults on patients, while Sanil was in the OR. Sarah was also helpful. She would offer to do things that Sanil hadn't even asked her to do. Even more telling, Deepak had told Sanil not to come in at 4 a.m. to pre-round. Instead, the team got their numbers (vitals) together during morning rounds at 6 a.m.

Afternoon rounds were different also. Over the last three days, the team had spent time at the end of rounds talking about how they could work more efficiently. So afternoon rounds had turned into a sort of collaborative problem-solving session instead of a "pimping" session where the chief asked rapid-fire questions of the intern, presumably to ensure that the intern had done the scutwork required to know every detail about patients.

When the night float team had been introduced in July, reformers like Deepak, Carl, and Sarah had each tried to use it to modify traditional sign-out practices. But reformers hadn't worked together, and, as I showed in the last chapter, defenders were able to block their individual efforts. Now with Carl, Sarah, Deepak, and Sanil all working together on a service, and with no defenders present to resist them, they could do as they chose. Afternoon rounds began to serve as what I call "relational spaces."[1]

In this chapter I will explore how, because of the way afternoon rounds historically had been conducted in the general surgery services at the three hospitals, these meetings served as relational spaces at Advent and Calhoun but not at Bayshore. At Advent and Calhoun, these spaces gave reformers in different work positions a forum for building a sense that change could be accomplished with newly developed task allocations. They allowed reformers to develop an identity that prescribed ways in which reformers in different work positions should behave with one another. Finally, the spaces facilitated the creation of frames justifying these new task and role expectations. Through the generation of this new relational efficacy, identity, and frames, reformers at Advent and Calhoun built a unified cross-position coalition that enabled them collectively to begin to challenge defenders of the status quo.

In the end, reformers at Calhoun were not able to maintain their coalition while those at Advent were, and in the next chapter I will explain why. But first, in this chapter, I will detail how Advent and Calhoun reformers initially built a cross-position coalition for change while those at Bayshore did not.

BUILDING OPPOSITION TO DEFENDERS

At all three hospitals, reformers did attempt to act against defenders. Groups of residents at the three hospitals often ate lunch together in the cafeteria. When defenders were not present, these cafeteria tables allowed for bonding and face-to-face interaction among reformers. Reformers at all three hospitals also often gathered to talk in the surgical resident call rooms or hospital hallways. Social movement theorists have called these kinds of spaces "free spaces" and have shown that they are important for allowing reformers to develop a sense of opposition to defenders.[2] In these free spaces, reformers at all three hospitals built oppositional efficacy, oppositional identity, and oppositional frames that led them to later challenge defenders.

Reformers built oppositional efficacy—a sense of hope that their efforts at collective action against defenders could be successful—by telling one another how they defied defenders and traditional practices.[3] For example, in a hallway conversation with several other reformers, one reformer chief at Advent told the group that one of the other chiefs (who was known by all to be "old school") had given him a hard time for not having his intern pre-round. The reformer chief said that he told the old-school chief, "They've been doing it this way in England for years." After hearing that story, a senior reformer smiled and said that he had been ragged on by one of the other seniors for doing "intern work" but continued to do it anyway. As reformers at the three hospitals began to tell each other stories about their defiance of defenders and traditional practices, they began to develop a sense of mutual loyalty and a belief that others would act with them to challenge defenders.[4]

Along with building solidarity, reformers at the three hospitals developed an oppositional identity by drawing boundaries between "us" and "them" and by defining defenders as adversaries who needed to be challenged.[5] They displayed a demeanor of "efficient resident" rather than Iron Man and called themselves residents who wanted to "have a life" rather than "live in the hospital." In their conversations with one another in free spaces, reformers began to construct themselves as "not old school" and to name old-school night floats and chiefs as adversaries who needed to be challenged. In one call room conversation with only female residents present, a senior Bayshore reformer said, "All of the old-school guys stay late for any case, no matter what time it goes. They've all got wives at home who are willing to 'stand by their man' regardless of never seeing him. But they need to be leaving those cases for the night float."

In addition to building a sense of oppositional efficacy and developing an oppositional identity, reformers at all three hospitals created oppositional frames by talking about the legitimacy of new versus old practices and discussing the unfairness of maintaining traditional practices.[6] When reformers met in free spaces, they created new ways of thinking about patient care (continuity of care by the team rather than by the individual) and resident education (learning by doing, but learning over a longer period).[7] For example, regarding resident education, one senior Advent reformer said at a reformer-only table during lunch:

> Some people say the interns won't see enough now that they aren't on call. But I found a journal article from a long time ago where attendings were complaining about exactly the same thing. Then it was because residents would no longer be on call every second night. . . . Even without taking calls, interns today are seeing more than they were back then because patients are a lot more acute now.[8] And even if they don't see everything this year, they will still be just as well educated by the end of residency.

THE BATTLE RENEWED

As they built up feelings of opposition vis-à-vis defenders, reformers at the three hospitals lobbied directors for additional support. As noted in the prior chapter, reformer chiefs had not alerted directors earlier to problems with the night float programs because they had not had anything specific to suggest regarding change and did not want to signal that they did not have everything under control on their services. But about five months after the introduction of the new programs, reformer chiefs in the three hospitals decided to enlist the help of the directors. Because of their mobilization with other reformers in free spaces, reformer chiefs now had a sense of oppositional efficacy, an oppositional identity ("not old school"), and oppositional frames ("continuity of care in team" and "learning by doing over a longer period of time") well worked out.

Reformer chiefs at each hospital successfully convinced the directors to begin publicly and emphatically reemphasizing their support of the new rule that night floats must accept handoffs from interns. This explicit reaffirmation by the directors led reformer chiefs and seniors to begin supporting handoffs more overtly and led interns to again begin attempting handoffs to defender night floats. As will be explained in further detail in chapter 8, interns who would be moving on to other specialties after one year in general surgery were particularly aggressive in handing off work to defender night floats.

Predictably, defender night floats resisted these renewed challenges. Reformers and defenders were again in an open confrontation with one another. One night float described his tactics for rejecting handoffs: "Joe [the intern] signs out stuff, like pre-ops. Before this, pre-ops had always been intern work. It is mindless busy work and all of us hate doing it. . . . So I started to show him that pre-ops were never my priority. A lot of it is non-verbal. Like when he says, 'Can you do these ten pre-ops?' I go, '*Sigh*. Yeah, sure.' Also, I try to do everything else before getting to them. Sometimes I just don't get to them at all."

When interns handed off routine tasks, defender night floats often "forgot" to do them. The combination of intern handoffs and defender night float resistance resulted in "dropped balls." Dropped balls were tasks left undone—usually tasks that were not critical to patient care but required for routine functioning of the service. Dropped balls caused trouble for the chiefs and attendings. While attendings were not involved in the details of the day-to-day work up on the patient floors, they certainly noticed when patients did not show up in their ORs as planned. Advent defender chief Matt Baker complained to me: "Rojas [the intern] signed out a pre-op to the night float and the night float didn't do it. So there I am doing damage control the next morning, running around trying to get this patient the right tests so he can go to the OR. Otherwise, [the attending] Wright's schedule gets all messed up."

At all three hospitals, defender chiefs responded to dropped balls by blaming specific interns for tasks that in fact were not completed by night floats. Bayshore chief Jim Nelson was outraged when he heard that a pre-op had not been done. Rather than blaming the night float, however, he blamed the intern. "Seniors have already done it [spent time during their intern year doing routine work like pre-ops], so why should they do it again? If I were a senior, I wouldn't want to do it."

In contrast, reformer chiefs responded to dropped balls by alerting directors to the problem. Defender chiefs countered by denying that night floats had purposely dropped balls. While far removed from the day-to-day work on the services, directors tried to find out the truth of the matter by talking with other residents. But at this early point, defender night floats were being supported by the powerful attendings and defender chiefs, and they continued to drop balls.

RELATIONAL SPACES AT ADVENT AND CALHOUN, NOT BAYSHORE

While change processes at the three hospitals were very similar for the first five months, they diverged once defenders began to drop balls. At Advent and Calhoun, reformers then engaged in a cross-position reformer challenge to pressure defenders to change their signout practices. At Bayshore, however, reformers in each position backed down as defender night floats dropped balls. This led to a divergence in handoffs across the three hospitals—interns at Advent and Calhoun began to accomplish handoffs in signout encounters, but interns at Bayshore stopped attempting handoffs altogether.

The difference in intermediate outcomes at Advent and Calhoun compared to Bayshore was associated with the availability of what I earlier called relational spaces. Afternoon rounds on reformer-only services at Advent and Calhoun became relational spaces because they were isolated from defenders and allowed for face-to-face interaction among residents from all work positions.

At all three hospitals, services were staffed in a rotating manner, such that every month there was a different constellation of residents (chief, senior, intern, and night float) assigned to each service. Most months, this constellation of residents included at least one defender, but there were a few months when services were staffed with reformers alone. But it was only at Advent and Calhoun that these reformer-only services had access to relational spaces. At these two hospitals, afternoon rounds on reformer-only services provided isolation from defenders because only residents assigned to the service were present in the room. Chiefs assigned to particular services had their favorite places to meet, such as conference rooms or quiet areas of patient floors, and, crucially, these areas were "private" in the sense that the staff could meet without being overheard by defenders. One Advent intern acknowledged that these spaces enabled him to express nontraditional thoughts more freely: "As an intern, there's no way I'm going to speak up in front of everyone. A lot of these guys are really against the changes. You'd be crazy to suggest it [in front of the whole group.] . . . When I was on Turner [a general surgery service] with Emily [reformer chief] and Chris [reformer senior], they were both very open to trying new things. So I felt comfortable suggesting things like how to handle pre-ops. We tried things and it worked well."

Advent and Calhoun afternoon rounds also facilitated a good deal of face-to-face interaction among reformers about broader matters than just patient care. Besides asking interns about that day's surgeries and appropriate care, reformer chiefs, seniors, and interns talked to one another about career plans and events in their personal lives. Thus, Advent and Calhoun afternoon rounds allowed residents on reformer-only services to spend what they called "downtime" together.

Finally, Advent and Calhoun afternoon rounds included members from each of the positions involved in the practice targeted for change. Typically, the chief, senior, and intern on the service attended afternoon rounds. Once the night float program was established, the night floats also often joined for at least some portion of afternoon rounds. The inclusive character of Advent and Calhoun afternoon rounds was important because any change to the signout practice would require the coordination and cooperation of residents from each of the work positions on the service.

Afternoon rounds at Bayshore did not allow for isolation, interaction, or inclusion. Even on reformer-only services, rounds were not held in "private" places but in an open surgical resident lounge; residents not assigned to the service were usually present. Moreover, afternoon rounds at Bayshore were limited to reporting on the status of patient plans. They were highly focused, and little spontaneous chatter marked these rounds. It wasn't as if residents at Bayshore did not fraternize with one another; it was just that because of historical routines, they did so in places other than afternoon rounds. Finally, Bayshore rounds were not inclusive. Either the chief or the senior attended afternoon rounds with the intern, but not both, and night floats were absent.

At Bayshore there were spaces, such as cafeteria tables, hallways, and call rooms, that provided reformers with isolation from defenders and allowed them face-to-face interaction with one another. But these spaces rarely included residents across different work positions on the same service. I never observed a situation where all residents on a reformer-only service ate lunch together or came together in the hallway or in a call room. Residents assisted surgeons in the OR during the day; it was extremely rare for all residents on the service to be out of the OR at the same time except during morning rounds, when time was tight.

Since the presence or absence of relational spaces seemed to me to be important, I examined my data carefully to explore what happened in the afternoon rounds as well as what happened in spaces such as call room and cafeteria conversations where reformers gathered, but not with everyone on their service. I coded data from the relational spaces and free spaces meetings I took part in at Advent and Bayshore. Since I did not do intensive fieldwork at Calhoun, I asked Calhoun residents in end-of-year interviews about what occurred during their afternoon rounds. I found that relational spaces allowed reformers at Advent and Calhoun to learn to work in new ways with one another. Without access to relational spaces, Bayshore reformers did not learn to work together in these new ways and so were never able to mount a cross-position challenge in the face of defender dropped balls.

RELATIONALLY MOBILIZING AT ADVENT AND CALHOUN

Relational spaces allowed reformers at Advent and Calhoun to build a sense of relational efficacy—an assurance that reformers in different work positions (chief, senior, intern, night float) would all work successfully to accomplish a new signout practice. Reformers at Advent and Calhoun built relational efficacy by collectively identifying task problems and jointly negotiating solutions during their afternoon rounds. For example, one day during afternoon rounds on the vascular surgery service, Margaret, an Advent intern, told others that because she was no longer arriving before morning rounds, she could not write her progress notes in the patients' charts before going to the OR. Later in the meeting Shelley, a senior, brought up another problem. She said she would like to help Margaret, but she had no way of knowing whether patient plans had changed since morning rounds. Since afternoon rounds included members from each of the work positions necessary to bring off a smooth signout practice, a forum for identifying problems was created.

With problems identified, reformers could now develop solutions jointly. Change in practice between two members of the team often required change by a third or fourth team member. In that same meeting, Diego, a night float, said that he could write the patient notes overnight so that Margaret would not need to arrive early to do so before morning rounds. But, he said, on nights that were unusually busy, he would not be able to get to the notes. Reformer chief Josh Levy said he supported the plan and suggested that when nights were busy, Margaret could write her notes later in the day. As to the problem of not knowing about changes in patient plans, Josh suggested that he could change his own practice and begin sending patient plan updates to the whole team rather than just to the intern.

Since team members frequently interacted with one another outside of afternoon rounds, they also improvised new solutions during the day by experimenting with solutions that had been collectively negotiated during afternoon rounds. These improvisations led both to the identification of new problems and to new ways of working together. These discoveries then came to light in afternoon rounds with all present. For example, as chiefs and seniors started to do more of the routine work usually done by interns, important information about patients was no longer being passed along normal channels and sometimes would get lost. A nurse, say, might ask an intern about what should be done for such-and-such a patient. But since the chief and senior had not told the intern what they themselves had done, the intern was not able to provide an answer for the nurse. When one chief noted that this was a growing problem, the residents discussed it in afternoon rounds and decided that whenever a resident on the service admitted a new patient, the resident would send everyone on the service an e-mail documenting key patient details.

At Advent and Calhoun, relational spaces also allowed reformers to build relational identity—a sense of self in relation to reformers in other positions. They did this by using language and demonstrating a demeanor in front of one another that supported the new task allocation. For example, reformers at the two hospitals referred to chiefs as "coaches" rather than "commanders." Seniors became "team players" rather than "wingmen." Night floats were "members of the team" rather than "stopgaps," and interns were "rookies" or "good prioritizers" rather than "beasts of burden" or "go-to guys."

A change in role expectations for one member often meant a change in role expectations for another. Once a senior started acting as a "team player" toward the intern by taking on some of the intern's routine work, for instance, he or she could no longer act as a "wingman" toward the chief by being available at all times as back up. Because all residents involved in the signout practice were present at afternoon rounds, they were able to negotiate these changes in interdependent role relations.

Reformers also elaborated new role expectations by behaving differently toward one another in reformer-only afternoon rounds than they did elsewhere. Reformer chiefs encouraged group discussion and decision making among members at all levels rather than holding the floor and issuing orders without explanation, as was the case on other services. Calhoun chief Lisa Sanchez explained: "If my intern missed something minor because he had signed it out, I'd be like 'You didn't do this, but it is OK.' But the old-school guys would be like 'What the fuck?' and then not talk to them." Intern Jane Morris at Advent described how a reformer chief, Emily, was "forgiving" when mistakes were made. "With other chiefs," she mused, "things I got yelled at for not doing are things I'm sure they never told me to do." She also mentioned that Emily talked to her more frequently and thoroughly than other chiefs, checking in midday and also sending a team e-mail, something almost unheard of on other surgical teams. The result was that there was less stress on the floor because there were fewer surprises.

Reformer seniors behaved differently as well. Instead of being aggressive and punitive with interns, seniors began treating them with apparent warmth and respect. While defender night floats did everything they could to signal their rejection of collaboration with the interns, reformer night floats consistently arrived a few minutes before 6 p.m., took time to ask interns' questions about patients when "running the list," and reacted courteously to unexpected delays. Interns, in general, responded by acting in a relaxed manner with reformers in other positions, although they continued to be subservient with defenders.

Reformer chiefs and seniors took on work they traditionally had not done. They presented themselves in front of other members on the service as willing to help the interns with any type of work. Donna, reformer chief at Calhoun, gave an example: "After evening rounds, I'd help the interns get the work on their scut list done. So if there was a discharge to do and a CT scan to check and a consent to get, we'd sit down and I'd say, 'OK, I'll go talk to the patient's family; you do the discharge.'"

As all members on the service helped one another during afternoon rounds, friendly and trusting relations among reformers in different positions began to develop. A team was created. Feelings of attachment with other team members led reformers to feel comfortable deviating from traditional role expectations. Because residents in all positions were present in afternoon rounds, each resident knew that the others were open to offering and receiving help across positions. Advent intern Lynn Wu remarked, "Now that I've gotten to know Chris [the night float], I know that he is being sincere when he tells me to hand off my pre-ops and post-ops. He's a good guy. I know that he's not going to go around telling other people that I'm 'weak.' . . . I also know that Josh [chief] knows that I'm handing off. That is OK with him."

In their afternoon rounds, both Advent and Calhoun reformers similarly created new sets of relational frames—justifications of new role relationships—in two ways. First, they explained why new task allocations were fair. For example, during afternoon rounds one day on the GI surgery service, Mary, an Advent reformer senior, told reformer chief Josh Levy, "Some of the night floats are grumbling that the interns are giving them attitude. They're refusing to take post-ops that came out [of the OR] before they arrived."

Josh responded by clarifying the role of the night float to everyone on his team. "The purpose of the night float," he said, "is to take the intern signout so interns can leave the hospital. It is unfair to the interns otherwise." Then he turned to Margaret, the intern, and told her, "You need to be signing everything out to the night float at 6. Otherwise, the longer you're here, the longer you're here. You will never get out of here if you don't do it."

As before, it was important that all members involved in the signout practice were present because a change in a frame justifying the tasks and role expectations for one position often required a change in frame for another position. In the example above, a change in frame for the night float (from "I've already paid my dues and have more important things to do" to "the purpose of the night float is to take the intern signout so the intern can leave") also required a change in frame for the intern (from "I need to be the first one here and the last to leave" to "the rules require me to leave the hospital"). Because both the night float and the intern were present for this discussion in afternoon rounds, both residents were able to hear these new, interdependent justifications.

The second way reformers improvised relational frames was rehearsing them in front of one another, thus developing frames that each came to believe in. In the interaction described above, the rotating night float for that night, Sally, was a reformer, and she reinforced the chief's frame when she said, "It's my job to take your signout. That's what I am here for. I have time." Here, again, it was important to have members in each position present so that they could all hear and commit to new frames. Calhoun reformer chief Betsy Shea was quite clear about this, saying she purposely discussed rationales for handoffs in front of the whole team rather than in individual conversations, in order to demonstrate her support for change to everyone on the service.

CROSS-POSITION CHALLENGES AT ADVENT AND CALHOUN

As dropped balls continued, challenges were risky not only for interns but also for reformer chiefs, seniors, and night floats. But reformers from each of these work positions at Advent and Calhoun continued to act collectively, drawing on what they were learning from one another. Interns attempted handoffs despite the risks to their reputation because in reformer-only teams they had discovered that the new system could work and that they could justify their challenges. Advent intern Nick Christakos told me, "Before I was just trying to do my work and was not so sensitive to how long it took. I'd drag my feet about calling the night float, and I'd be down there [in the pre-op area] doing pre-ops before calling them. . . . But now I've realized that it's the night float's job to do pre-ops. And that . . . our [the interns'] priorities should include getting out on time."

Reformer seniors helped interns with routine tasks because they saw themselves as team players and because they had developed reciprocal friendship bonds with interns. Reformer night floats overtly accepted hand-offs because it was "their job" even though there was clearly no personal benefit to them from taking on more work. They were sanctioned by some of their peers for doing so, but as a night float reformer said, "Some of the night floats are way too focused on what the interns aren't doing instead of on the fact that we get to go home at night now on every rotation except this one. One scut rotation is a small price to pay for getting to work eighty hours a week instead of one hundred."

Similarly, reformer chiefs promoted handoffs by handling "minor snafus" (which defenders called "dropped balls") and not denigrating the interns involved. Apparently they did this because they had seen that it was possible to effectively carry out the new signout practice as long as other residents on the service were willing to take on nontraditional tasks. Gradually, they had come to see themselves as "coaches of teams" rather than as "commanders of beasts of burden." Calhoun chief Donna Russo noted: "Some people are old school and like to bring the hammer down on the interns when the night floats don't do something overnight. Just like in the military. In that situation, I think it's just as much a problem with the night float as with the intern. I'll tell both of them how I think we can do things better. But I don't go around screaming at everyone."

NO RELATIONAL MOBILIZATION OR CROSS-POSITION CHALLENGES AT BAYSHORE

As I noted earlier, there were no relational spaces at Bayshore. Reformers at the hospital were not able to create the assurance that fellow reformers in different work positions on the service would complete the tasks required to successfully use the new signout practice. Nor did they develop new role expectations and justifications for them. Without building relational efficacy, identity, and frames for the new practices, they were unable to create and sustain a cross-position challenge in the face of defender dropped balls.

In free spaces such as hallways, call rooms, and cafeteria tables, I sometimes saw Bayshore reformers identifying problems to one another and even talking about solutions. But reformers who congregated in these free spaces often did not work on the same service with one another. Without the presence of reformers on the same service from each of the work positions, reformers were not able to gain a broad perspective on the problems they faced, nor were they able to work out and negotiate solutions with one another. In one call room conversation I heard, two senior reformers on different services, Julie and Elena, discussed the problem of interns staying late. They were able to identify the causes of the problem and to come up with potential solutions:

> JULIE: The interns are still staying late every night. I think we need to improve this. The night float should take over the duties early enough so that others can go home. We need to make a habit of rounding earlier. Then if the intern is swamped, we can help.
>
> ELENA: The problem is that the way it is now, the intern can ask the night float, but there is only a 40 percent likelihood that it will get done. Sometimes the night floats don't know what is supposed to be done. The interns have to take care to make sure the night floats know what is going on.

But neither Elena nor Julie was able to try out their solutions. Elena was staffed on a reformer-only service at the time, but none of the other reformers from the service were present for this conversation. There was no forum where reformers on the same team could all work together in the absence of defenders to come up with potential solutions that they could support.

Occasionally new practices were attempted. But things fell through the cracks because there was no space for negotiating joint solutions to problems. One night Rob, an intern on a reformer-only service, had several patient admissions left to do. During signout he told David, the reformer night float, about a lab test the chief had ordered for a patient with a colon infection. Rob ran through the list of patients and ended his signout by saying, "If you could draw labs, it would be great." He meant for David to draw labs on the patient with the colon infection, but David misunderstood, thinking he was being asked to draw labs on only the newly admitted patients. The next morning, the reformer chief was upset that the labs on the patient with the colon infection had not been drawn. This was a dropped ball. At Advent and Calhoun such problems had occurred as well; however, team members had talked through such communication mishaps during reformer-only afternoon rounds and tried to develop ways to ensure that necessary information was properly passed on and understood by all. At Bayshore, no such group discussions occurred.

In free spaces such as hallway conversations at Bayshore, I sometimes saw reformers on a reformer-only service trying to behave in new ways by offering help to one another. But again, since they did not all gather as a group, reformers in each work position on the service did not have the opportunity to try out new interdependent and helpful roles vis-à-vis one another. To be sure, reformer chiefs and seniors helped interns and saw themselves as "being nice," but the change did not stick.[9]

Interns who handed off routine tasks to reformer night floats blamed themselves if the night floats did not complete the tasks. In the end, they did not expect night floats to do these tasks even though they asked. Critically, they did not work with the night floats to solve problems. To illustrate, one reformer night float, Heather, told Charlie, an intern, that she was happy to write progress notes in the patients' charts overnight so that he could take care of his more urgent tasks before leaving the hospital. One night, however, Heather was not able to write these notes. The next day when Charlie came in, he discovered that the notes were not done. There was no time for him to do them between answering pages and going to the OR. So he had to take the progress notes to the conference and try to write them there. They didn't get done until the end of the day.

When similar problems had occurred at Advent and Calhoun, they had been addressed in the afternoon rounds meeting. It was accepted that notes could be written later in the day by the intern if the night float had been too busy to get to them. Reformers at Advent and Calhoun had developed the expectation that the night float was a "member of the team." He or she was responsible for progress notes, but it was assumed that this could not be an inflexible rule; exceptions must be allowed. At Bayshore there was no such change in role expectations. Charlie blamed himself for what he perceived to be a failure to do his own work. Because the chief expected Heather to be a "stopgap" rather than a "member of the team" and because she saw Charlie in the traditional role of a "go-to guy" rather than a "good prioritizer," she never asked him why he did not get the notes completed. She ended up blaming Charlie as well even though she was sympathetic to change.

Although reformers at Bayshore did justify new task allocations or role behavior to one another as they talked throughout the day, these discussions were typically dyadic. There were no opportunities to get collective agreement about what needed to be done and why it should be done in a new way. I heard reformer chief Helen James on a reformer-only service at Bayshore tell an intern, Andrew, that it was necessary for the senior to do some routine work during the day so that Andrew could leave at the end of his shift. But without the presence of that reformer senior, there was no opportunity for Helen to persuade him that the new task allocation was justified. Nor was there an opportunity for Andrew to check and see whether there was a consensus among other service members around the justification offered by Helen.

At Bayshore, reformers never stood up to defenders, and reformers continued to worry that handoffs could not occur without dropped balls. Reformer chief Bikram Singh said, "Elena was trying to help the intern during the day, but it didn't work. Things inevitably fell through the cracks, even though Elena was trying to be helpful. . . . It may be that it's just not possible in surgery for this to work."

Without a new relational identity outlining new role expectations, Bayshore reformer seniors saw themselves in the traditional way, as "wingmen" to the chiefs. Reformer night floats continued to see themselves as "stopgaps" handling emergencies overnight rather than as team players who helped interns with routine tasks. Without relational frames justifying new task allocations, Bayshore interns believed that routine work was "their job." Moreover, it was their "own fault" if they were not fast enough to finish tasks by the end of their shift. Bayshore reformer chiefs and seniors felt that routine tasks were "intern work" rather than work that they should be taking on to ensure that the intern did not have many tasks left at the end of the day. Because they had not developed these new relational capacities, Bayshore reformers in all positions quickly backed down when balls were dropped.

*   *   *

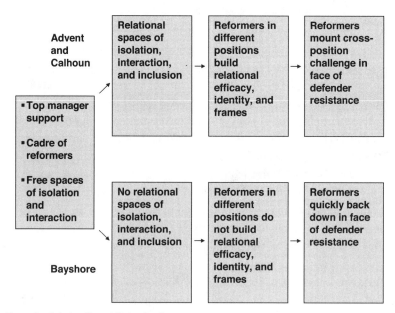

Figure 6.1. Relationally mobilizing for change

At all three hospitals, reformers built a sense of opposition vis-à-vis the defenders, but only at Advent and Calhoun did reformers engage in relational mobilization vis-à-vis one another. What clearly differentiated Advent and Calhoun from Bayshore was the existence of relational spaces at Advent and Calhoun—spaces that were physically isolated from defenders of the status quo, that facilitated face-to-face reformer interaction, and most critically, that included reformers from all the work positions involved in the practice targeted for change. At Advent and Calhoun, reformer chiefs, seniors, night floats and interns built relational efficacy, identity, and frames within these spaces that enabled them to mount cross-position challenges to defenders in the face of dropped balls. At Bayshore, reformers did not have relational spaces within which to mobilize and did not mount cross-position challenges in the face of defender resistance. Ultimately, they failed to change the traditional signout practice (figure 6.1). But as the next chapter shows, only at Advent were reformers able to maintain their challenge long enough to force defenders to change their traditional signout practices.

7

Countermobilizing
for Resistance

Paul Robertson, defender chief at Advent, was furious. He had just finished operating on a patient when Don Mueller, a vascular surgery attending, came into the OR and informed him that Mrs. Wilson, the patient Mueller had been scheduled to operate on next, had been canceled because she had a yeast infection. Mrs. Wilson had already had anesthesia and was in the OR for a 7:30 case when they discovered it.

Paul groaned and apologized for not catching this, but as soon as Mueller left, he threw down the gray notebook in disgust, strode to the OR door, flung it open, and dragged the wheeled patient gurney, with his sedated patient on it and the nurses clinging to the other end, out with him. "This is unacceptable," he fumed. For the second time this week, an operation had had to be canceled due to a "dropped ball." During morning rounds just two days earlier, Adrian, the intern, had told Paul about a different patient whose operation had to be postponed because he couldn't get heparin. As Paul was wheeling his patient toward the PACU (post-anesthesia care unit), he told me: "Adrian should have known sooner and done something about it. This would never have been accepted in the past. The problem is that there is no fear now. In the past, you just got it done. It is maddening. So weak! Mueller was being nice. This is a major screwup! The intern should see every patient twice a day. I have thirty patients to see in an hour. The juniors on the floor are my eyes and ears. It is unacceptable and it will be dealt with."

Paul yanked the front of the gurney through the swinging door into the PACU and pulled it into one of the empty patient post-op bays. "[The intern] is in the OR right now. But as soon as he gets out, we're going to have a come-to-Jesus talk," Paul declared as we left the PACU to go up to the floor. But by the time we exited the elevator on the fifth floor, Paul seemed somewhat defeated, no longer convinced that his "come-to-Jesus" talk with Adrian would solve the problem. His voice heavy with frustration, he lamented the loss of the old days in surgery: "There was more esprit de corps in the past. You'd camp out in the fifth-floor lounge during an Iron Man weekend. In between calls, you'd hang out and have pizza. You'd hang around the hospital and do whatever came up. It was like battlefield buddies are the best. Everyone pulled together. These people were your family. You had no outside interests." He went on:

> Advent is known as a really tough program. When I'd go to conferences, people would say, "You're at Advent? Oh my God." It has been one of the best, the hardest places to get into. Only the toughest, strongest could survive. We traditionally have six spots and would only go down as far as six or seven on our rank list in the match. Things have definitely changed. Now the interns are a bunch of softies. These new interns came in expecting to get out at 6 (p.m.). They interviewed last year asking about the hours change. They have a different mindset. I expected to work straight through for seven years. People who didn't want to do it self-selected out. This year everyone on the interview trail asked about work hours. Was it going to happen or not? Only one guy didn't ask about it, and I wanted to take him. Everybody else asked about lifestyle. So now we have a bunch of part-time surgeons. A bunch of wusses!

Like other defenders, Paul was blaming the interns for dropped balls, disregarding the fact that pre-op work such as detecting patient yeast infections or ascertaining heparin requirements before surgery was now the official responsibility of the night floats. "Could the night float have done anything differently to prevent this?" I asked.

"No!" Paul retorted. "I expect the interns to get it done. This is not shift work. They are getting a lot of sleep. Six to six is not the right way to go. You can postpone the pain and dump it on the next guy [the night float]. But it is your [the intern's] patient. The night float is not part of the team. He is covering thirty people. Something is going to slip through the cracks."

When interns handed off routine work like pre-ops, defender night floats often resisted it passively by neglecting to do the work overnight. The frequency of dropped balls increased. This was infuriating to Paul and the other defenders at Advent and Calhoun. They blamed the failure of the system on the interns who handed off to the night floats. Defenders were convinced that the chief and senior reformers supporting the interns were "ruining surgery."

By attempting handoffs in the face of resistance, interns and other reformers struck at the very heart of the Iron Man's world. Handoffs challenged not only the traditional practices the defenders were skilled in using but also the cultural demeanor they had perfected, the positional relations that afforded them high status in the profession, and the underlying meaning system that supported the status hierarchy. In short, reformer-defender interactions were cultural and political contests in which the legitimacy and authority of the Iron Men and the institutions that supported them were confirmed, denied, or left in doubt. To the Iron Man, such challenges were not to be taken lightly. Their own legitimacy and authority were at stake.

I was not surprised that the defender chiefs at Advent and Calhoun were outraged by the actions of the reformers. But it was interesting to me that the frequency with which defenders used labels like "weak," "soft" and "wuss" to denigrate them increased once reformers started collectively challenging defenders. It was clear that the battle was entering a new phase. Before, defenders had pushed back on individual handoff attempts by "teaching" the interns and even "beating" them in front of others with warnings about how handoffs led to poor patient care and inadequate resident education. But now that reformers at Advent and Calhoun were collectively challenging defenders, different strategies had to be found.

And so defenders turned to new, less subtle strategies of retaliation, strategies they apparently thought would be more effective in the surgical social world than accusing someone of not delivering good patient care or of not being well educated.[1] They began to label their enemies "weak," "softies," "part-timers," "wusses," "pantywaists," "girls." Defenders at both Advent and Calhoun used divisive countertactics to try to split the reformer coalitions at their respective hospitals. In this chapter I describe these tactics and explain why the coalition of reformers at Calhoun allowed itself to be divided and eventually defeated while Advent reformers successfully faced down countermobilization.

SIMILAR DIVISIVE COUNTERTACTICS AT ADVENT AND CALHOUN

As explained in the previous chapter, at Bayshore there were no spaces available where reformers with diverse identities and work positions could interact with one another apart from defenders. Thus Bayshore reformers were not able to create a unified collective with one another across subgroups. Defenders pushed back on handoffs, and Bayshore reformers capitulated within several months in the face of these arguments.

In contrast, as noted, at both Advent and Calhoun, spaces did exist where male and female reformers from different work positions could mobilize themselves apart from defenders. By organizing to attempt handoffs in the face of resistance, reformers presented a sustained collective challenge to defenders. In response to this collective challenge, defenders at both Advent and Calhoun turned to harsher strategies of retaliation than they had used in the first several months of the resident year. Their countermobilization involved a three-pronged attack, each prong designed to divide the reformer coalition at their hospital: (1) negatively labeling reformer practices, (2) denigrating particular reformers, and (3) recruiting reformers into the defender camp.

The first countertactic the defenders used was negatively labeling reformer practices. Defenders devalued reformer practices by arguing that they were associated with the stereotypical negative female resident characteristics of "weak," "soft," and "caring about personal life rather than being committed to work." One female resident noted, "The guys who are against the changes are saying that surgeons have always been the marines and now they are becoming soft."

Similarly, a Calhoun chief asserted, "All of this stuff about [imitating a high female voice] 'Ooooh, I'll do this for you. Ooooh, let me help you get out of here'—it's bullshit. The interns need to learn to do it themselves." He insisted that reformer practices were followed only by those who were "soft" and "weak."

Defenders also labeled reform practices "feminine" by associating them with stereotypically feminine behavior. For example, they suggested that the reform practices were used by those who wanted to work "part time." One defender chief noted: "When you're an attending, it isn't a 9 to 5 job, so I think that you're fooling yourself if you think that you're going to be able to work eighty hours. The attendings work more than eighty hours a week here. So if you think that you're gonna go through this process acting like a part-time doctor, I just don't think that's compatible with a career in surgery." A Calhoun female reformer noted that males who opposed the change in work hours were "always rolling their eyes and making snide comments about the female chiefs hanging out at home." At Advent, too, defenders often told stories of female reformers leaving the hospital at the end of their shift.[2]

By using a high voice when they talked about the reform practices, emphasizing how these practices required "helping" behavior, and calling those who used the new practices "part-time workers," defenders associated new practices with stereotypical femininity.

The second countertactic defenders used was to denigrate particular reformers. For example, a Calhoun defender stated bluntly: "There is a change of attitude in the freshman class. . . . You have to build some toughness into your character, and that's lacking. Now they're softies." "Pantywaists" and "girls" were other terms defenders used to denigrate male reformers who used the reformer practices such as sharing work with other kinds of care providers. One defender said, "The interns are a bunch of pantywaists. When I was an intern on cardiac, I never left [the hospital]. Two of us covered it all. Now they have three residents, a [staff surgeon] in the cardiac ICU, and six PAs on the floor. I took vein all the time. They never do . . . [With disgust] It's all part of the kinder, gentler residency."

One defender told me with evident distaste about a male reformer who had been leaving the hospital at the end of his work shift and talking about life outside of the hospital: "I had one intern who [at the end of his shift] was like 'Gotta go. I have to leave, I have a picnic.' I kid you not, that's what he said, 'I have a picnic to go to. I'm going to stay for a little and then I have to go.'" A layperson may not think of going to a picnic as a feminine act, but to defenders, going to a picnic was beyond the pale, a clear sign of softness, of prioritizing the feminine domain of home and hearth over the masculine domain of the organization. In the world of surgery, putting personal life ahead of work was a breach of some magnitude.

The third countertactic the defenders used was recruiting reformers into the defender group. After shaming the reformers, defenders let them know what they would need to do to be forgiven. One defender chief told me how he had handled a male intern who was engaging in the reformer practice of leaving the hospital at the end of his work shift as the formal rules required:

> I had one intern who, when he first got onto the service, was weak. . . . He was trying to leave at 6 and get other people to do his work. So I beat on him. I would quiz him in front of a group of the patients. I would put him on the spot and say, "So what did the CT show on Mr. Jennings?" . . . I was pissed off. I wanted [the intern] to understand with some negative reinforcement that it wasn't acceptable. . . . In two days, he started to get it. He cracked. It was like an epiphany. Then he said, "I'm worried that I am not doing a good job," which from a guy who has gotten all A's through [elite university] and has never been told that he has done a bad job at anything in his life, was intensely gratifying, and he said, "What am I doing wrong?" and I told him in pretty clear terms what I wanted him to do, and for the last week that I had him he started to do it.

SUBSEQUENT DIVERGENCE AND ALTERNATIVE EXPLANATIONS

While both relational mobilization and the use of divisive countertactics were similar at Advent and Calhoun, member action in the two hospitals diverged over the course of the year. At both hospitals, internal reformers engaged in reform practices early on. But at Calhoun, by the end of the year most residents reversed their early practices and resisted reform. In contrast, reformers at Advent continued to engage in reform practices through the end of the year. Interns handed off work to the night float whenever they had such work left to do at 6 p.m., and chiefs supported them in their efforts. Moreover, chiefs at Advent who had been defenders at the beginning of the year had begun by the end of the year to adopt these reformer practices too.

How can we explain these different outcomes?

Before detailing why the reformer coalition was maintained at Advent and not at Calhoun, it is important to consider what we might expect the answer to be given existing social movement theory. In explaining coalition maintenance, social movement theorists point out that reformer groups are not monolithic but are composed of subgroups from varying backgrounds, each having different grievances. Coalitions form but are often fragile and difficult to sustain.[3] Research suggests that four key factors affect the maintenance of a reformer coalition across subgroups: (1) similarity in goals, (2) common reformer frames and practices, (3) high political opportunity, and (4) high countermovement threat.[4]

But each of these factors was more or less identical at Advent and Calhoun. First, at both hospitals, reformers in different subgroups (e.g., other-specialty residents, female residents, egalitarian men) banded together to fight for change. While reformer goals were not the same across subgroups at either Advent or Calhoun, the goals of each subgroup—improving the position of other-specialty residents, improving the position of women, and increasing time for personal life—were the same at each hospital. Thus, differences in goals across subgroups cannot explain why Advent reformers kept their coalition together and Calhoun reformers did not.

Second, as noted in the last chapter, through their work with one another in relational spaces, reformers at both Advent and Calhoun successfully built a set of common reformer identity claims, frames, and practices. Reformers referred to themselves as "progressive residents," "team players," "complete doctors," and "surgeons with a life." They emphasized that "it is possible to achieve continuity of care in the team," that "men and women can both be good surgeons," that "it is important to learn by reading and working in the clinic in addition to learning by operating," and that "residents learn better when they were well rested." And they built a common set of oppositional practices. They hung out together in mixed-gender groups and told stories of "stupid macho old-school" behavior. They shared routine work across different positions. They told stories about their personal lives while at work. They took time for floorwork. They talked about surgical diagnoses and postsurgical problems as well as about operations. And, critically, they went home at the end of their shifts. These identity claims, frames, and practices were inclusive of the key concerns of each of the reformer subgroups—interns, other-specialty residents, female residents, and male residents. Thus they allowed reformers to build a "we" across subgroups. Yet this was true at both Advent and Calhoun.

Third, political opportunity existed at both hospitals. The larger medical world was pushing for change, and the door was open to reformers. Directors at both hospitals provided important resources for reform. Because of these political opportunities, defenders could not retaliate against the reformers in any obvious or draconian way—by, for instance, ejecting residents from the program. Defenders were forced to use indirect and less obvious tactics.

Finally, there was high countermovement threat at both Advent and Calhoun. High countermovement threat is a unifying force, because it reminds and helps persuade reformers in different subgroups that they must work together to defeat a common adversary. At both hospitals, defenders countered reformer frames with their own frames—for example, arguing that handoffs were bad for patient care and resident education. Defenders organized by building a collective identity of "old school" residents and by sharing tactics with one another. And they tried to create political opportunities for themselves by enlisting the support of attendings in covertly repressing reformers. Since the social context of both opportunity and threat was quite similar at Advent and Calhoun, it cannot explain why Advent reformers sustained their coalition while Calhoun reformers did not.

In sum, social movement theory as currently constructed does not account for the divergent outcomes at Advent and Calhoun.

SUBGROUP THREAT AT CALHOUN BUT NOT ADVENT

I argue that the difference in outcomes at the two hospitals was associated with different degrees of subgroup threat posed by female residents at both, a threat that existed even before the new night float programs were introduced. This subgroup threat included two components: career threat and identity threat.

First, regarding career threat, during the year the night float programs were initiated, there were more female residents among the resident leaders at Calhoun than at Advent. At both hospitals, as at most hospitals across the country, most years there was a much smaller number of female chief residents than male chief residents. While about 45 percent of the intern classes were historically composed of female residents, female residents exited the residency program at a greater rate than male residents, so there were many fewer female residents at the top of the hierarchy than at the bottom. Historically, only about 10–15 percent of the chief resident classes at the two hospitals had been composed of female residents. But as chance would have it, during the year the night float program was introduced at the two hospitals, the percentage of female chiefs at Calhoun (38 percent) was higher than historically at Calhoun and also higher than at Advent (14 percent). Because men had historically been dominant, increasing numbers of women in high-status positions at Calhoun led female residents to be perceived as a career threat by the male residents, while they were not perceived as a threat at Advent.

Second, in addition to posing a career threat to male residents by occupying senior positions, female residents at Calhoun posed an identity threat to male residents by acting like Iron Men. At both hospitals, female residents challenged the behavioral distinctions between male and female residents in some ways. For example, at both places female residents wore the same surgical scrubs as did the male residents, and like the male residents, female residents in both hospitals told stories of idiotic medical residents, unflappable staff surgeons, annoying nurses, and "train-wreck" patients (patients who were seen to have no chance of living when they arrived). Female residents strode rather than walked through the hospital, paged jokes back and forth to other residents, and lobbied their chief residents for more difficult cases.

Yet I was struck by the fact that female residents at Calhoun used a wider range of masculine practices than did those at Advent. In terms of dress, in the important space of the operating room, Calhoun female residents wore surgical caps like the ones worn by male residents (and like those shown on TV), while at Advent the female residents wore "shower caps" like the lower-status nurses. Similarly, Calhoun female residents, in my observations, did not wear any jewelry or makeup, while Advent female residents did. In terms of demeanor, Calhoun female chiefs told about giving their interns nicknames, while at Advent it was only the male chiefs who had that prerogative. Calhoun female residents told of going out drinking, while Advent female residents told me they rarely did so. Calhoun female chiefs told of "throwing bones" (assigning cases that were officially above the required resident year) to their interns, while Advent female chiefs did not. Finally, Calhoun female residents recounted episodes of having aggressively "told a staff surgeon to move over" in the operating room so that they could take charge in the operation, while Advent female residents reported avoiding even being suspected of doing this.

There were certain masculine acts that even Calhoun female residents did not engage in. For example, Calhoun female residents reported that they did not tell war stories of OR prowess the way the male residents, did nor did they aggressively pimp (rapidly quiz) interns or lose their tempers. However, overall Calhoun female residents appeared to engage in many more masculine acts than did Advent female residents. Because they acted masculine in so many ways, female residents at Calhoun threatened the masculine identity of male residents.

RESPONDING TO DIVISIVE COUNTERTACTICS AT CALHOUN AND ADVENT

At Calhoun, in the context of high subgroup threat, defenders' pressure proved too much for male reformers and they responded to divisive countertactics by abandoning the reformer cause. Even the two male chiefs whom residents reported to have been publicly strong supporters of the work-hours changes when the night float program was introduced were demobilized by defenders. A story is worth telling here.

As the end of the resident year approached, chiefs voted on teaching awards for the attendings. The three female chiefs and the male chief who had initially been the most vocal male reformer all voted for one staff surgeon who was known to take time with the residents, teaching both during surgery and outside the OR. The remaining four male chiefs voted for another "very macho" staff surgeon. Then the male chief who initially had voted for the first surgeon sent an e-mail to all the chiefs saying that he had changed his vote, specifically so that "the women wouldn't win."

The female chiefs were outraged. One female chief, brown hair escaping from her ponytail and pale after a long day in surgery, took me into an office with a closed door. In a voice full of defeat, she recounted the incident to me:

> So the one guy who was on our side said verbatim, over e-mail, "Well, I don't like him either but I'd rather see the girls suffer. Women shouldn't be in surgery anyway." So he changed his vote and made it 5–3. And then that e-mail was followed by the other guys saying "Ha-ha, we won" or whatever. Eight people all e-mailing, and the final e-mail was from one of the guys who wrote and said: "You women, you lost, and let's face it—surgery is a man's sport." Which was the last line of his e-mail. And not a single one of the guys, in my class or any other class, because of course everybody heard about it, said that it was unacceptable. Not a single person stood up and said, "That's not right." It was just accepted.

After this incident, the female chiefs told me, the interns, male and female, began once again to stay on past the end of their shifts. Several of these interns reported to me that when they stayed late in the hospital, rarely were they involved in patient care that the night float could not handle. Instead, they said, they were doing paperwork to maintain their reputations as "strong" residents who did not hand off work. They simply gave up. Sam, a male intern, aptly summed up the rule that prevailed in the work lives of residents at Calhoun: "Even though the female chiefs told me to go home and not to come in on Saturday, I still came in. . . . Reputation is everything in this program, and everyone knows who's here and who isn't."

As implied by Sam's remarks, female chiefs at Calhoun continued to resist the defender's countertactics. In contrast to the other reformers, female chiefs chose to engage in collective action to improve their female chief group's status rather than to try to exit into the more highly valued defender identity group. Several reasons seem to account for this. First, the female chiefs still questioned the legitimacy of the defender's status. They didn't buy into the "old school" values of machismo, individualism, and hierarchy. Second, the female chiefs believed the boundaries of the defender group to be impermeable. Although defenders claimed that a female resident who resisted change could be "one of the guys," female chiefs were unconvinced: "It's easy to be 'one of the guys' when you are a junior resident, because you are doing all of the scutwork for the senior male residents. But once you are [a chief] and you are the one giving orders, they no longer want you as one of the guys. . . . It's like 'That's so cute that that girl is doing well; she is my junior high school student.' But this is one of the few times when you can go straight from being the slave to being the competitor."

Third, female chiefs were under less pressure to abandon their cause than were other female residents. The female chiefs were in their last year of residency. They had already secured fellowships for the following year. While their reputations with attendings were jeopardized during the year that they pushed for change, they were less dependent on these attendings than were interns and seniors who would remain at Calhoun.

Finally, based on their experience to date, female chiefs were convinced that, no matter what they did, they would not have the same professional opportunities as did the men. One female senior explained:

> I think women will always be at a disadvantage. When I started as an intern, I thought the problem was not my generation—if we just got women into surgery, everything would be all right. Now, I realize my generation is no better. There is a barrier there that just doesn't exist for men. In surgery, you have to run things exactly how you want them to be. That will always open up the door to people thinking that you are a bitch, which is the standard defense against a strong woman. So one of the ways you get around that is you develop good relationships with people and you try to do it as nicely as you can. . . . I guess you do it the same way that the less privileged, less favored groups have always done it, which is—you just have to be very good.

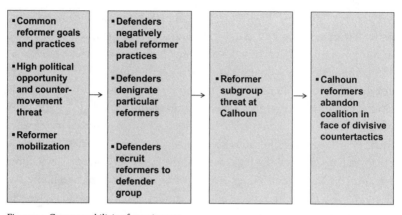

Figure 7.1. Countermobilizing for resistance

In sum, at Calhoun male reformers and all female reformers but the chiefs backed down in the face of defender tactics. Female chiefs sustained their activism in the face of these tactics, but largely because they felt they had little to lose. They were on their way out of Calhoun, a bit wiser perhaps as to why the change had failed, but still supportive of it.

While Calhoun reformers allowed defenders to divide their coalition, Advent reformers did not. Because the subgroup threat at Advent was low, male reformers there did not experience concerns about loss of male privilege. Male reformers at Advent were less concerned than those at Calhoun about being seen as feminine or being left out of the Boys' Club. One male reformer chief remarked to me over lunch: "The old-school guys like to say that handoffs are weak, that we are all becoming soft. I don't buy it. Unless we do things differently, surgery is never going to change."

In the end, Advent reformers in all subgroups stuck by the senior female reformers in the face of divisive countertactics.

*   *   *

At both Advent and Calhoun, defenders of the status quo used divisive countertactics to attempt to divide the reformer collective.[5] They negatively labeled reform practices, denigrated particular reformers, and recruited reformers to the defender group. The responses to these tactics differed between Advent and Calhoun. What differentiated the two responses was the greater initial subgroup threat at Calhoun. As noted in figure 7.1, the threat to traditional male positions and behaviors led male reformers at

Calhoun to abandon the coalition to protect their status and its rewards. At Advent, the privilege of male reformers was not under threat from female reformers. There male and female reformers maintained their coalition in the face of divisive countertactics and were able to sustain their challenge long enough to force defenders to change the traditional signout practice. How they did this is the subject of the next chapter.

8

Collectively Disrupting

What caused defenders at Advent to buckle under reformer pressure? Some insight can be gleaned from an anecdote told to me by an Iron Man attending when I asked him why he changed his tune about the work hours issue. He told me that his abrupt about-face was sparked by a specific incident. In animated fashion, he said that he began to go along with the change in April when he heard a story (which I later heard from several other defenders in essentially the same form as he related it to me) about a phone call between Bob Goodwin, Advent's Director of Surgery, and Bill Manning, Advent's highest status surgical attending and a legend in the department. Apparently, Goodwin was halfway through a meeting when his secretary put a call through. Manning was on the line. "Goodwin," Manning was alleged to have barked, "I just had another dropped ball. This is ridiculous. Night floats need to take intern handoffs and it's never gonna happen the way you currently have things structured."

And that was it, just the one phone call. Yet when the story of that phone call swept through the hospital, everyone who heard it was startled. For here was Manning not simply complaining one more time about the eighty-hour workweek; instead, he actually seemed to be abandoning his opposition to handoffs. Manning had been a vocal and powerful defender who had been speaking out against the new work hours ever since Goodwin announced the impending change fourteen months earlier. Now Manning was on the phone reversing his position and saying he was ready to go with the change. Why?

In this chapter, I will explain how reformers at Advent successfully changed the long-standing signout practice by not only relationally mobilizing and standing up to countermobilization but also effectively engaging in a process I call "collectively disrupting." Reformers interfered with daily activities and, in doing so, compelled defenders to accommodate themselves to a new practice and legitimate it so that it became judged by key audiences at Advent as beneficial, understandable, and morally correct.[1]

Interns who would be moving on to other specialties outside of general surgery after they had trained there for one or two years were critical to the acceptance process. Because these other-specialty interns would be pursuing careers outside of general surgery, they were transient reformers. Since they would not become general surgeons, they were less committed to general surgery roles and accounts, and their careers were less vulnerable to the potential long-term damage of defender attacks. For these reasons, they were willing to wage the most confrontational battles against defenders.

Other-specialty interns were not unique to Advent; they were present at Bayshore and Calhoun as well. In fact, Bayshore had the highest percentage of other-specialty residents (51 percent, versus 27 percent at Calhoun and 35 percent at Advent). But since reformers at Bayshore had not built a cross-position coalition through relational mobilization, other-specialty interns there had immediately backed down at the first sign of dropped balls. And since reformers at Calhoun had not maintained their cross-position coalition in the face of countermobilization, other-specialty interns there had retreated too soon to make a difference. Only at Advent did reformers both build and maintain a coalition. By doing so, they created an opportunity for a collective disruption process at Advent. Aggressive activism by the outsider other-specialty residents clearly depended on something more than having little to lose; they were aggressive because they felt they had something substantial to gain.

INTERFERING WITH DAY-TO-DAY ACTIVITIES

General surgery interns at Advent acted as reformers in the face of defender resistance, but they attempted change in less risky ways than did other-specialty interns. When defender night floats were moderately resistant, general surgery interns attempted handoffs, but when these night floats vigorously resisted, general surgery interns backed down. In contrast, other-specialty interns at Advent put their heads on the proverbial chopping block, no matter how staunchly they were resisted, refusing to back down in the face of night floats' active handoff rejections. They ignored beatings given to them by their chiefs for dropped balls, and they shrugged off defenders' negative labeling and stigmatization. By sticking their necks out to engage in adversarial challenge in the face of aggressive retaliation, these other-specialty interns disrupted the day-to-day functioning of the general surgery services.

One of the ways that other-specialty interns interfered with day-to-day activities was to essentially force defender night floats to do the work they were required to, even in the face of active handoff rejections. One evening I was following Anand Roy, one of the staunch defender night floats, when Michael Walker, a urology intern, signed out. Michael handed off two pre-ops, and Anand rolled his eyes. Michael then handed off a post-op check on a patient who had had an appendectomy. Anand tried to reject it, pointing out that the patient had been out of surgery for three hours and thus implying that Michael should have done the post-op check himself.[2] Michael explained that he had been in an intern conference.

ANAND: We always blew those things [conferences] off.

MICHAEL: It was mandatory for us.

ANAND: Yeah, it was for us, also.

MICHAEL: [Program director] told us to go.

ANAND: [sighing] Well, he's the boss.

After he finished handing off the post-op check, Michael tried to give Anand the stack of index cards tracking each patient on the service so that Anand could update them overnight. Anand balked, saying he didn't need the cards. The two wrangled a bit about whether using cards was the best practice. Anand refused to take them. Michael shrugged and left. But rather than backing down in the face of Anand's rejection by taking the cards home with him, as he would have done before the mobilization at Advent, Michael swung by the call room and left them there for Anand. Anand later told me that Michael was weak to have handed off the pre- and post-ops to him:

It's a different mentality than before. Before you didn't hand off anything to anyone. You crossed all of your t's and dotted all of your i's before you left the hospital. And you would never sign out anything to someone higher than you. It was considered a sign of great weakness. . . . One thing that has considerably changed is that people are just willing to sign out things. It's a huge shift in mentality. We always thought poorly of it. Now I'm like, fine, if this is what they want to do then it will be this way. But I wouldn't do it if I were them.

The next day I caught up with Michael to ask him why he handed off the pre- and post-ops. He knew that he had made Anand angry, he said, but he didn't care. "If you didn't ever sign out post-ops, you'd be here late every night doing them. I consider the pre-ops fine to sign out also. He's here all night. It's his job. Things are often not ready [pre-op charts do not arrive until late in the day]. There are very few things you can do at 11 a.m. The labs are not back yet and the pre-ops are not ready. That was my time that was free yesterday."

Michael clearly had embraced the reformer frame that the night float was part of the team. Rather than blaming himself for not having completed all the routine work on the service during the day, Michael thought it was fair to expect the night float to take care of whatever he had not completed by 6 p.m. At this point in the year, Michael's interpretive frames were similar to those of his fellow other-specialty interns. They felt they had something substantial to gain, and little to lose, by disrupting daily activities. Like his peers, Michael was spending only one year in general surgery, and therefore he had little stake in learning to comply with general surgical norms or respecting a hierarchy he would not be climbing. As one general surgery intern bluntly put it: "What does Michael really care about what general surgery thinks about him? There is a stigma attached to signing out pre-ops and post-ops. [Unlike Michael,] I'm trying to build a reputation for the next seven years."

Nick Christakos was another other-specialty intern. Like Michael, he followed the new rules and handed off work to night floats no matter how hard they tried to make it for him. Even though these defender night floats never paged him when they arrived, he looked in all the key resident hangouts until he tracked them down. Nick told me that he didn't feel bad handing off things that were due or that happened after 6 p.m. If night floats treated him decently, he was flexible in return. But if they badgered him, he stood his ground. Defender night floats would hem and haw, roll their eyes, call him weak, trying everything they could to get him to yield, but Nick made a point of not backing down. Because he saw reformer chiefs and seniors continue to press for change in the face of defender countermobilization, he felt that change had a good chance of succeeding. And because he would be leaving general surgery at the end of the resident year, he was willing to stand up to defenders in ways that general surgery interns, whose career interests were at stake, were not.

Another way other-specialty interns disrupted day-to-day activities was to ignore the beatings their chiefs gave them for "dropped balls." A typical strategy of staunch defender night floats was purposely to "forget" to do any routine tasks handed off by interns that were not critical to patient care but required for the routine functioning of the service—and they were particularly "forgetful" when interns handed off the tasks despite their attempts to dissuade them. Such dropped balls, of course, caused trouble for the chiefs and attendings, but one of the staunch defenders, Daniel Cohen, justified his actions by pointing out that the patients were not his patients: "Some of these guys like Nourazar [an other-specialty intern] expect me to treat their patients overnight. I refuse to do it because I don't know them. I don't advance diets, I don't change meds. I don't do any fine-tuning overnight. I don't feel comfortable doing it. And it's not just that. It's also that I don't have any claim on these patients. I don't like tinkering with other people's patients. So I don't."

Defender chiefs cooperated with this defender night float strategy, blaming the interns rather than night floats for dropped balls and delivering beatings to shame the interns into submission. One night, Fred, a defender night float, failed to put a patient on certain nonurgent home medications. The next morning at rounds, rather than blaming Fred, defender chief Matt Baker yelled at Joe Nourazar, the intern. When I talked with Joe later that day, he seemed anything but beaten down. In fact, he justified his handoffs, telling me that he was in the right and that he was confident handoffs would work well if they were supported by other team members. These frames, identity, and sense of efficacy apparently spurred him to continue to attempt change in the face of defender resistance. "In the beginning, I felt bad about signing out," he said. "The night float members would be at dinner bragging that they still had a few hours before the interns were ready to sign out. . . . After being with a few helpful night float members and chiefs, I began to look at it differently. Now I feel like I'm not asking for a favor. . . . The night float is part of the team."

Other-specialty interns were more willing to ignore defender chief beatings because they were not dependent on senior defenders' judgments for access to longer-term resources such as fellowship recommendations. For example, other-specialty intern Miguel Rojas told me about an incident in which Fred, a defender night float, hadn't updated the patient cards that Miguel had left for him. During morning rounds, Miguel's defender chief, George Farrell, had asked Miguel about nonurgent lab results on one of the patients. Miguel had said that he didn't know the results, that they had come back overnight and Fred had not written them on the card. "You're the intern," George had shouted. "That's your job. You need to know every detail about your patients!" Miguel smiled at me and said, "George wasn't too pleased. But either we have a night float system or we don't, and as long as we have one, I intend to use it." Miguel was apparently not worried about the possibility that George would gossip about him and sully his reputation.

A final way that other-specialty interns disrupted day-to-day activities was to shrug off defender labeling and stigmatization. For example, on the vascular surgery service, other-specialty intern Stephanie Lewis consistently handed off at 6 p.m. and left the hospital. Her defender chief and senior and the rotating defender night floats gave her a tough time. Sometimes it was subtle, or at least relatively nonconfrontational: they ignored her, joked about her behind her back. Other times it was not so subtle: they made cutting jibes about her during afternoon rounds. Stephanie was aware that they were purposely excluding her, but at this point in the year, she took this in stride:

> They all get dinner together and don't invite me. So I'm not really friends with that core group. I've ended up finding friends in other places. I've made friends with some of the nurses and some of the people from other specialties. You need to have friends here because you are here so much. . . . It hurts when I don't feel part of things and when I get yelled at. But I try not to take it personally. . . . I just want to be done with this.

Stephanie wasn't willing to stop attempting handoffs in hopes of winning the approval of the defenders. So although it wasn't pleasant, she took defender stigmatization as a matter of course and looked ahead to better times when she would no longer be part of the general surgery residency program.

Like Stephanie, most other-specialty residents found friends "in other places"—and most often these friends were other other-specialty residents. While they did not formally make agreements about what they would and would not do, they did end up telling each other how they had handled altercations with defenders and supported one another in the face of aggressive handoff rejections. One afternoon as I followed Adrian Galanis checking patients on the floor before afternoon rounds, he told me, "I hang out with Nick and the other-specialty residents. We don't really belong here. We're one step lower than the other interns. . . . We sign out a lot of stuff, but that is the way it is supposed to work with night float. We've all had confrontations with the old-school guys over it. They make nasty jokes about us. They insult us to our faces. They don't let us do the good cases. But we get together, and we laugh about it. . . . We'll be gone soon."

Other-specialty residents' mutual support was critical in the face of belligerent behavior by the defenders. One night I was out at the Alibi, the corner bar near the hospital that was frequented by Advent residents on Wednesday nights. People were sitting at tables, here half a dozen men in work boots and dusty jackets loudly telling stories, there two couples in conversation, and in the middle, standing in circles talking, surgical residents, some dressed in scrubs, others in street clothes. The waitress, a young brunette in a shirt hanging off her shoulder, hurried to and fro carrying a tray laden with glasses of beer. A short time after we arrived, Nick and Joe, two other-specialty interns, came in. Peter, the defender senior on Nick's service, was standing near the door. "Oh, look who's here," Peter said sarcastically. "I'm sure you made sure everything was tied down tight before you left."

Later that night Peter came over to Nick again, and this time it was easy to see that he was three-parts drunk. He lurched against a table where Nick was sitting with Joe and another other-specialty intern, Brandon. Peter knocked over a glass of beer as he pressed a finger into Nick's chest. "I make your life difficult on purpose, you know," he said. "And, I'm going to do whatever I can to break you. It's gonna make me happy to crush you like a bug."

There was complete silence at the table. When Nick didn't answer, Peter turned slowly around and walked away. "Shit," Joe said to Nick. But Nick shrugged it off: "What an asshole."

FACILITATING DEFENDER ACCOMMODATION

While other-specialty interns played the most confrontational role in change by disrupting routine activities on the surgical services, reformer chiefs, seniors, and night floats played an important supportive role: they informed attendings and directors about the reformer nondisruptive model of handoffs and offered defenders a solution that would allow them to meet their most important goals. As noted in chapter 6, directors had played a hands-off role in the day-to-day implementation of the changes. Although they had been actively involved in the development of the night float teams before the beginning of the resident year, once the teams were introduced they turned their attention elsewhere, and it wasn't until about five months later that, at the behest of reformer chiefs, they stepped back in the ring by reinforcing their support for the changes. Attendings had been more involved in day-to-day resident activities, gossiping about reformers with defender chiefs and seniors in the PACU and withholding teaching from reformers in the OR. But even attendings had been uninvolved until this point in the resident interaction up on the floors, which was where signouts occurred. Now dropped balls had led both the directors and attendings to pay more attention to the residents' methods of caring for patients.

Reformers began to make the new reformer model of handoffs visible. Reformer night floats did this by drawing attention to the fact that not all night floats were dropping balls. They suggested that some night floats were "lazy" and were "giving all of the night float members bad reputations." One morning on his way out of the hospital, for instance, reformer night float Ben Davis ran into attending Frank Conrad coming out of the brightly lit coffee shop next to the front lobby. Frank waved Ben over. "What's going on with you guys overnight?" he asked. "I've had more dropped balls in the last month than in the last two years."

Ben replied. "Some night floats are irresponsible. There is stuff they know they shouldn't let slide and they do. Like ordering labs for the morning, updating cards, making new cards for admits. No intern is going to tell on them [for not doing it]. But it is just the right thing to do. . . . Some people doing this have such a sense of entitlement. Like 'I shouldn't accept sign-out at 6 [p.m.] when I'm the one covering overnight.' . . . We feel like it is going to reflect poorly on the rest of us."

Like reformer night floats, reformer chiefs made a point of explaining to attendings how handoffs could be accomplished effectively as long as chiefs, seniors, and night floats were supportive of change. When attendings expressed anger about lapses in patient care, reformer chiefs pointed out that dropped balls were not a necessary outcome of handoffs. They argued that there were not problems with patient care in handoffs between interns and reformer night floats whenever the chief, senior, and night float on the service were willing to work in a less hierarchical manner by taking on routine work.

Reformer chiefs had access to the directors through their weekly director-chief meetings. They made sure that the directors knew that there was both a good and a bad model for handoffs. Reformer chiefs had not begun to tell directors sooner about specific night floats who were refusing to take intern handoffs because the relationship between the directors and the reformers was a formal one, and officially reporting misconduct of fellow residents was unacceptable under the surgical norm of "covering the backs" of fellow residents. Traditionally, "covering the backs" of fellow surgical residents had protected surgical residents who made errors by not revealing them to medical doctors, patients, or anyone outside the surgical profession.[3] Since speaking negatively to directors about fellow residents transgressed a traditional surgical norm and broke resident solidarity, reformer chiefs did not feel comfortable doing it until dropped balls had created a crisis situation that negatively affected the directors and attendings.

In one director-chief meeting, reformer chiefs drew attention to the difference between positive and negative handoffs by talking about problems associated with a few rotating night float members:

REFORMER CHIEF JOSH LEVY: Daniel Cohen was on last night and he was terrible. He takes all of his calls from the bunk.

REFORMER CHIEF EMILY SCOTT: Sometimes when he was on overnight, he wouldn't even be there when I got there at 6 am. Anand Roy is a problem, too.

DEFENDER CHIEF HARI AGARWAL: I haven't had any problems with them.

REFORMER CHIEF EMILY SCOTT: It's a personality thing. Some of these guys, like Carl Johnson or Susan Hill, are great. They're good about taking intern handoffs, and when they're on overnight I never have any problems.

In addition to telling attendings and directors about a nondisruptive model of handoffs, reformer chiefs, seniors, and night floats offered defenders a solution that would allow them to meet their most important goals. Until early April, defenders at Advent had resisted change largely because handoffs conflicted with time-honored traditions. But defenders had other reasons for resisting handoffs as well. Attendings wanted to avoid having to communicate with a greater number of people about their patients because they feared handoffs would disrupt continuity of care. Defender chiefs wanted to act as commanders molding the new interns into "workhorses" and were concerned about relying on multiple residents to accomplish routine work. And defender night floats wanted to minimize their overnight workload and avoid taking on the kind of work that would negatively affect their status.

By aggressively attempting handoffs in the face of dropped balls, other-specialty interns had created a situation where resisting handoffs did not allow defenders to accomplish all of their goals. By resisting handoffs, attendings did achieve one goal—they avoided communicating with multiple people—but they failed to achieve another, continuity of care for patients. Defender chiefs found themselves in the same bind. By resisting handoffs, they were acting as commanders transforming interns into "workhorses," but they were not getting routine work accomplished. If they encouraged interns to hand off work, they would not be acting as true "commanders" of would-be Iron Men. But the chiefs also felt duty-bound to be "go-to guys" for the attendings by ensuring that all work on patients was done overnight.

In the end, weighing choices in light of their understandings of situational exigencies, Iron Man chiefs decided that their obligation to the attendings was stronger than their obligation to teach interns in traditional ways. Defender chief Paul Robertson explained: "If something doesn't get done, as the chief resident, you are responsible. You are it. The attendings expect you to take care of everything. . . . You are expected to know everything and do everything, or you get a beating for it."

Night floats found themselves in the same situation. By resisting handoffs, they minimized their overnight workload. But their reputations suffered as a consequence of dropped balls. When defender night floats Daniel Cohen and Anand Roy learned that their names had been brought up in front of the directors at the weekly director-chief meeting, they were furious that their reputations had been sullied.

By disrupting daily activities, other-specialty interns had created a situation where defenders had to become open to new ways of doing things. And reformer chiefs now proposed a new way. The staunchest defender night floats were the rotating seniors in position 3, working only once or twice a week. In contrast, position 2 on the night float team was filled by seniors who, like those in position 3, did not want to do routine work, but they worked six nights a week for an entire six-week rotation. Reformer chiefs reasoned that they could replace the recalcitrant rotating seniors in position 3 with a designated intern currently assigned as a "day float" across the general surgery services. The reformer chiefs brought this up in several different weekly meetings with the directors:

REFORMER CHIEF DEEPAK PATEL: The [rotating night floats] are a problem. Anand Roy was on last night. When I asked him why he didn't make up a new card on an admit that came in overnight, he said he didn't know they were supposed to do the interns' work.

REFORMER CHIEF EMILY SCOTT: We need to get rid of the [rotating night floats]. We could move the intern day float into that position and it would solve the problem. [Emily was suggesting that they replace the rotating night float member with the intern currently assigned to a "day float" position, working on different general surgery services depending on which were busiest at the time.]

After several meetings, the directors agreed to the reformer chiefs' plan and proposed the idea to the attendings. The attendings initially resisted it because they did not want to lose the extra help with coverage during the day that the day float provided. However, as the problems caused by dropped balls continued, the failure to agree on a solution created a crisis for attendings. Presented with the evidence of successful handoffs among reformers, ten and a half months after the introduction of the night float program and five months after dropped balls had become a topic of concern, the attendings agreed to have the intern from the day float position replace the senior in the rotating night float position.

Interestingly, this same solution was available at Bayshore and Calhoun—in all three hospitals there was an intern serving in a day float position who could have been moved to replace the rotating night float. Indeed, reformers at Bayshore and Calhoun had suggested this solution to the directors, and the directors had talked to the attendings about the possibility. As they had initially at Advent, attendings at Bayshore and Calhoun resisted this idea because they did not want to lose extra help with coverage during the day. The solution was not adopted at Bayshore or Calhoun because reformers there had not collectively challenged defenders in the face of dropped balls. As noted in chapter 6, reformers at Bayshore did not engage in relational mobilization and so did not collectively challenge defenders at all. As recounted in chapter 7, reformers at Calhoun did not maintain their solidarity in the face of countermobilization. Since reformers at these two hospitals had not maintained their collective challenge in the face of dropped balls, there was no "crisis" at Bayshore and Calhoun to force the attendings to accommodate reformer demands.

LEGITIMATING NEW PRACTICES

Soon after this change in staffing occurred at Advent, general surgery interns joined other-specialty interns and began to attempt handoffs; night floats across the board began to accept handoffs. However, it was not only the change in staffing that led to the acceptance of change. While the new structure of the night float team restored the traditional hierarchy on two of the four teams covered by night float members (now interns were signing out to interns on two of the four teams), the handing off of routine work still violated the traditional surgical hierarchy on the other two teams, where interns were signing out to seniors. And of course, handoffs still violated the traditional Iron Man identity and the traditional "continuity of care" and "learning by doing" frames.

In order for handoffs to become accepted practice at Advent, they needed to be seen as desirable, proper, and appropriate within the socially constructed system of roles, authority relations, and accounts at the hospital. It was prior defenders who now legitimated the new practices. They did it in three ways—by using reformer frames and identities to justify handoffs and portray handoffs as a valued way to behave, by recrafting sanctions to make it in the best interest of night floats to accept handoffs, and by teaching new frames, identities, and rewards to newcomers at the point of their initiation into the organization.

Defenders who had argued that handoffs were detrimental to patient care now began to suggest that handoffs were not really a problem. For example, previous defender chief George Farrell said, "I was definitely concerned that with all of the handoffs patient care would suffer. But it is fine, because people are extremely conscientious." These defender chiefs now suggested that although the interns might learn more slowly, they would still learn all they needed to know by the end of residency. Prior defender chief Matt Baker said: "It might be that they can't put in chest tubes and lines themselves. But that's a technical thing that can be taught in their second year. That is not what makes a good intern or a good doctor. I'll teach them lines and chest tubes next year."

Prior defenders also sought to persuade others to accept handoffs by borrowing reformer-created identities. One of the ways they did this was by selectively using characters and plots from the world of sports. They talked about night floats as "team members" rather than "wingmen," about chiefs as "coaches" rather than "commanders," and about interns as "rookies" rather than "beasts of burden." In the old cultural narrative, interns were expected to come in as "beasts of burden" and to be molded by "commander" chiefs into midlevel "wingmen" en route to becoming "commanders" themselves. In the new narrative, interns would come in as "rookies," learn to be "team players," and one day become "coaches" themselves in charge of training new interns.

Surgical residents historically had used sports terms to emphasize endurance and competition. When psyching up one another to do a tough case in the OR, they would say, "Put your game face on." Now, in contrast, they drew on sports narratives to validate collaborative behavior. Accepting handoffs was now a way to "be a team player," and doing pre-ops was a way for a senior to "take one for the team."

This change in vocabulary had an important consequence. Residents were able to accept and even value their new collaborative activity by rejecting the stereotypical female metaphors they had used to characterize it earlier ("weak, soft") and reinterpreting it using sports metaphors ("coach," "team," "player," "rookie"). One advantage of the sports narrative—and perhaps this helped facilitate its broad acceptance—was that it was consistent with the highly valued Iron Man persona. Thus, whether conscious or not, reformers' construction of their activities as consistent with sports narratives was central to marshaling later defender support for new forms of action.

In addition to using reformer frames and identities to portray handoffs as the valued way to behave, prior defenders recrafted sanctions to encourage handoffs. They began to badmouth night floats who dared to resist. In all but two of the signout encounters I observed once the change in staffing was made, night floats smoothly took work from the interns. In the two cases where this did not occur, it was the senior resident Peter Martin, serving in position 2 on the night float team, who did not accept handoffs. He passively rejected one handoff and avoided volunteering for another. Peter's resistance soon became common knowledge. He told me that he thought it was "weak when interns handed off their work." But he also told me that Matt Baker, a prior defender chief, had told him that he needed to "be helpful." It was difficult for Peter to maintain his resistance. Before the rotating night floats were replaced with the intern, Peter had been part of a larger group of night float defenders. But now that this rotating group of residents had been replaced by a single night float intern—and moreover one who supported change—if Peter continued to drop balls he would be highly visible as the only person resisting handoffs. Not surprisingly, Peter backed down and began to smoothly accept handoffs.

The new support of the prior defenders also made it easier for interns to attempt handoffs. One general surgery intern reported, "I've started handing off. . . . I used to think of night float as not part of the team, that they were stopgaps just to get the patients through to the next day. Now even the old-school chiefs assume that the night float will do it. Before, as the intern, I would think, 'It's my fault if it doesn't get done.'"

A final way that prior defenders legitimated handoffs was by teaching new frames, identities, and rewards to newcomers at the point of their initiation into the organization. As they began to use handoffs regularly in signout interactions, Advent residents acted out new understandings in particular situations. However, in order for these new understandings to shape future action, residents needed to externalize understandings produced by particular residents in particular circumstances so that they became taken for granted as "the way we do things."

New understandings at Advent were extended beyond particular work interactions when members narrated them to other members. One formal opportunity to do so was the chiefs' orientation presentation to the incoming interns regarding their expectations for the coming year. At this presentation, instead of telling the interns that they should not hand off work to the night float resident, chiefs stated that interns needed to work with night float members as a team. One chief's PowerPoint slides said, "Night float needs to take responsibility and be accountable. Night float shouldn't drop the ball."

Another narration opportunity occurred a few weeks later in July, when the interns moving into their second year of residency taught the incoming interns the tricks of the trade and provided ready-made accounts for the new signout practices. They communicated the same understandings that had been narrated by the chiefs at orientation. For example, a former intern now moving into his second year as a general surgery resident told a new intern assigned to the intern night float position, "You'll do a lot of pre-ops on night float, especially at the beginning of the year because the interns won't get to them. I always make cards for the next day when I do pre-ops because I'm looking it [patient data] up anyway." Through the narration of new understandings such as these, residents communicated new institutions that would shape future actions.

Residents also communicated new roles to incoming recruits. Rather than acting as "working machines" who "don't eat and don't sleep," interns were to act as "well-organized" and "efficient" workers who "know how to prioritize tasks." Instead of completing tasks in the order they were listed on the patient roster, interns were taught to "think about what tasks are most important for you to complete yourself and which should be handed off to the night float." I also heard prior defenders use new language to talk about themselves. For example, in their June orientation presentation to the new interns, new chiefs who had been defender fourth-year residents the previous year emphasized that night floats were "part of the team."

Finally, attendings, chiefs, and seniors who had previously defended the status quo now rewarded interns and seniors who attempted and accepted handoffs with good cases, extra teaching, and inclusion in their high-status group. Thus the incoming interns were immediately taught that attempting and accepting handoffs was valued behavior. Prior interns moving into their second year of residency communicated what was socially defined as an exterior and objective reality. As a result, the new interns internalized the understandings and used them in different times and places to shape their actions.

There were still a few diehard defenders at Advent, diehards such as senior Peter Martin, who continued to believe that traditional practices were best even as he reluctantly complied with the new practices. But now it was the defenders who kept their identity secret from others. Peter told me in private, "Now even the old-school guys are supporting handoffs. I still think it's wrong. I still think the interns aren't going to be as well trained if they do it. But I'm not going to advertise that. I'm going to do what I'm told." This suggests that the legitimation process may continue at Advent as each generation of residents communicates the emergent reality to incoming recruits. As one resident said, "Come back here in five years and this will be a totally different place. People won't even believe it when we tell them how it used to be."

WORK HOURS, EDUCATION, AND PATIENT CARE AT ADVENT

How did these changes affect resident work hours, education, and personal life outcomes at Advent? How did they affect patient care? Since hours were not being officially tracked, it was not possible to use timesheets to measure the reduction in work hours. And experience with hours tracking at other hospitals suggests that given all of the pressures on residents to misreport their hours, timesheets are not an accurate measure anyway. Observation

Interfering with Daily Activities	→	Facilitating Accommodation	→	Legitimating New Practices

Who	• Transient reformers	• All reformers	• Prior defenders

How	• Refusing to back down in the face of new practice rejection	• Publicizing an alternative model	• Selectively using reformer frames and identities
	• Ignoring "beatings" received for activity disruption	• Offering defenders a solution that allows them to achieve their most important goals	• Recrafting sanctions to punish traditional practices
	• Withstanding insults and stigmatization		• Teaching new frames, identities, rewards to newcomers

Figure 8.1. Collectively disrupting

is more reliable. My tracking of signout encounters showed that by the end of the year, interns were consistently handing off all tasks left to do at the end of their day to night float residents. Moreover, end-of-year interviews I conducted with Advent members in private suggested that residents had dramatically reduced their work hours.

In these end-of year interviews, some residents noted that they were still concerned about educational outcomes. But an analysis of ABSITE (American Board of Surgery In-Training Examination) test scores (which are designed to measure resident knowledge each year) shows that scores were rising, not falling. Regarding patient care, in my end-of-year interviews with prior defender residents and attendings they expressed surprise that the changes had had no negative impact. Attendings felt that some minor things such as the ordering of noncritical tests were "falling through the cracks," but even they did not think that these missteps negatively affected patient care. And residents uniformly reported that the quality of their work and personal lives had dramatically increased since the night float team was introduced.

*   *   *

At Advent, reformers collectively disrupted traditional practices and forced the legitimation of new practices (figure 8.1). Other-specialty interns, who were both less committed to traditional roles and frames and less dependent on defender rewards than general surgery interns, played a critical role in this process. Once it became clear that reformers at Advent had a chance of accomplishing change, other-specialty interns began to actively interfere with day-to-day activities. They refused to back down in the face of defender rejection of handoffs, ignored verbal beatings received in response to dropped balls, and shrugged off insults and stigmatization. Reformer chiefs, seniors, and night floats played an important supportive role in the collective disruption process by informing attendings and directors of the reformer model of handoffs and offering defenders a solution that would allow them to achieve their most important goals. After prior defenders had accommodated a change in practice, they used their reputation and high status to legitimate it so that handoffs became the accepted practice at Advent.

Conclusions and Implications

Many thought that the problems associated with patients' and residents' rights would be solved by regulating the work hours of residents. It was just a matter of time, they felt, before all hospitals would move to enforce the regulation. And in the years since this regulation was introduced, hospitals like Advent have indeed changed their work hours, successfully implementing the new regulations. But the path to change has not been as easy, as successful, or as widespread as optimists had hoped. The regulations took effect in 2003, yet in the intervening years the ACGME has had to take action against hospitals that have continued to violate them. Even more disturbing, there is enough evidence of inaccuracies in residents' reports to suggest that many of the hospitals that are thought to be complying with the regulations in fact are not.[1] These data suggest that Bayshore and Calhoun are not the exceptions but the norm. The puzzle this book set out to solve is why some organizations attempted and accomplished change and why others—similar in many respects to those that did change—resisted and failed.

SINCE 2004—REFORM REVISITED

When I left the field at the end of 2004, hospitals were having a difficult time reducing resident work hours. A *JAMA* study based on anonymous resident reports showed that at the end of the first year of regulation, interns were working more than eighty hours per week in 67 percent of hospital general surgery departments.[2] This particular study has not been repeated since, and no other anonymous, broad-spectrum study is available.[3]

Yet evidence suggests that hospitals are still struggling to implement reform. In 2007, pressured by reformers who argued that the initial work-hours regulation introduced by the ACGME had not been effective in solving patient care and resident safety problems, Congress directed the Institute of Medicine (IOM) to study the issue. The IOM committee heard testimony from groups on both sides of the work-hours divide and issued a 2008 report that recommended additional limits. The report noted that while "there are simply too few data to reliably estimate the extent to which errors in performance by fatigued residents affect patients and cause them harm, . . . there is considerable scientific evidence that 30 hours of continuous time awake, as is permitted and common in current resident work schedules, can result in fatigue. There is also extensive research that shows that fatigue is an unsafe condition that contributes to reduced well-being for residents and increased errors and accidents."[4] The committee recommended that hospitals institute a new protected sleep period of five hours, a "nap," inside the hospital during any work shift beyond sixteen hours in duration. It also suggested increasing time off between shifts and recommended that other agencies in addition to the ACGME monitor compliance.[5]

The response to the report from defenders and reformers alike was negative and uncompromising, though for different reasons. Defenders from medical professional associations such as the American College of Surgeons retorted that additional restrictions on residents' duty hours would compromise both the continuity of care for patients and the education of residents.[6] Reformers from organizations such as Public Citizen, the Committee of Interns and Residents, and AMSA said the new restrictions did not go far enough. They argued that the problem would not be solved until the national government, not the profession, monitored residents' work hours.[7] They scoffed at the idea of a five-hour period of protected sleep, noting that "enforcement of current guidelines has been lax and enforcing guidelines on sleep within shifts will be even more difficult."[8] They suggested that work hours would not truly be reduced until hospitals were given funds to hire ancillary staff and fined for work-hours violations.[9]

Regardless of where one stands on the desirability of the regulation, it is hard to disagree with the reformers' arguments about what would be required to improve compliance with it. Even so, I would argue that even their recommended changes do not go far enough. The reformers' assumption is similar to the macro-institutionalists' view that it is environmental pressures, organizational characteristics, and top-manager commitment that drive institutional change. In the preceding chapters, I have provided evidence that a view of institutional change that focuses primarily on such macro-level factors ultimately fails. In this concluding chapter, I summarize how collective combat occurred on the ground inside the three hospitals, draw out the implications of this study for our theoretical understanding of institutional change, and advance several concrete recommendations for those interested in implementing medical reform in surgery and elsewhere.

COLLECTIVE COMBAT INSIDE THE HOSPITALS

To recap, the impetus to change work hours was initiated outside the three hospitals I studied. A social movement composed of patients rights' and residents rights' reformers sparked a sense of moral outrage about resident work hours among the general public and drew the public's attention to the fact that surgical residents were working 100–120 hours per week. These long hours, it was argued, posed risks to both patients and residents. Dramatically, reformers called for Congress to establish federal regulations limiting work hours for residents.

Not unexpectedly, a countermovement formed. Those opposed to the change in hours argued that reducing resident work hours would actually lead to an increase rather than a decrease in the number of patient errors. Shorter resident work hours were dangerous, they claimed, because they resulted in more handoffs of work between residents, increasing opportunities for error.

The countermovement failed to persuade the general public. Reformers won the macro-level battle, and the medical profession preempted the threat of outside control over daily medical practice by regulating itself. In spring 2002, the Accreditation Council for Graduate Medical Education (ACGME) announced new regulation limiting resident work hours to eighty per week.

In theory, the new regulation had teeth because the ACGME could deny accreditation to programs that did not comply. Reimbursement for training residents and resident board certification depended on this accreditation.

Directors of the three surgery departments I studied responded by introducing similar compliance programs that made use of night float teams. Predictably, surgical attendings were outraged. Making change would require violating valued roles, long-standing authority relations, and deeply held beliefs. Department directors did, however, have allies in their residency programs. While about a quarter of residents strongly resisted change, residents who had strong alternative social identities or low-status positions in surgery became early advocates for reform.

But as directors tried to implement the new programs, anti-change residents and attendings defended the status quo by organizing with one another, preempting interns' attempts to use the night float program, rejecting handoff attempts when they were made, and punishing residents for the handoffs that did occur. Change attempts were consequently thwarted, and residents continued to work long hours, as they had before the new programs were introduced.

The defenders' initial success in blocking change at all three hospitals was a professional rather than organizational matter. Interns, as newcomers to the profession, wanted to prove their worth to colleagues such as night floats, chief residents, and attendings with whom they would be assigned to work in the future. Interns cared less about their hospital's rules than about their colleagues' standards for appropriate conduct and how they could gain access to further training and social acceptance.

The defenders' response generated a reformer counterresponse. Reformers built cross-position coalitions to collectively challenge defenders. They created new ways of working by identifying problems and jointly solving them. They put forth novel language and acted in new ways to develop a new set of roles. And they justified their new tasks with one another across positions. This posed a formidable challenge to the old guard. To the degree that the reformers were successful, it was because they had access to places where they could develop relationships with one another safe from the interference of defenders—places that facilitated face-to-face interaction and included all members involved in the practice targeted for change. At Bayshore, where no such spaces existed, no collective challenge emerged.

Once it was apparent to defenders that a collective challenge was being mounted, they tried to divide the reformer coalition. The success of the defenders' divide-and-conquer tactics depended largely on the strength of the initial subgroup threat present in the organization. At Calhoun, subgroup threat was strong because high numbers of women were in senior positions the year of the change and the female residents acted like Iron Men. Here defenders had an easy time dividing the male-female reformer coalition by threatening the status of male reformers. They negatively labeled reformer practices, denigrated particular reformers, and recruited reformers to the defender group. As a result, all but a few reformers at Calhoun backed down and surrendered. At Advent, where the subgroup threat was weak, reformers successfully resisted these countertactics and, as a result, managed to maintain their coalition for change.

While change ultimately failed at Bayshore and Calhoun, reformers were victorious at Advent. It was a hard-fought process, resting in part on collective disruption. Advent reformers interfered with day-to-day activities and forced defenders to accommodate new practices if they were to meet their own goals. The key contextual factor here was the presence of transient reformers—interns who were not pursuing a general surgical career. Because they were seeking careers outside of general surgery, they were less vulnerable to the potential long-term career damage of defender attacks and thus were willing to defy defenders. While transient reformers were present in all three hospitals, they were critical at Advent because only there had other reformers sustained their coalition long enough to create problems for defenders.

Table 9.1 details the collective combat processes used by reformers and defenders at the three hospitals, the mechanisms that composed these processes, and the local resources that facilitated them.

THE TWO LEVELS OF INSTITUTIONAL CHANGE

These findings challenge three central ideas in our current understanding of institutional change. First, in the predominant view, reform is driven by macro-level actors external to the organization. Change occurs because institutional entrepreneurs question existing norms and logics, professionals seek to increase their power, social movements interpret events as representing new threats to or opportunities for the realization of their goals, or interest groups challenge a profession's monopoly. My focus on the micro level suggests that while institutional entrepreneurs, professions, social movements, and interest groups may be necessary for institutional change, they are not sufficient. There must also be reformers located inside organizations who fight for change against internal defenders. At least in the hospitals I studied (and I suspect almost everywhere), powerful organization members resist attempts to change long-standing work practices both because these practices further their material interests and because new practices challenge a cultural style they have perfected, authority relations that afford them high status, and a meaning system that supports this cul-

TABLE 9.1. Collective combat processes inside the hospitals

COLLECTIVE COMBAT PROCESSES	FACILITATING RESOURCES	CHANGE MECHANISMS
Defending stability	Professional alignment of reformers	Preempting compliance program use Preventing program use Punishing program use Organizing with other defenders
Relationally mobilizing	Relational spaces	Building relational efficacy Developing relational identity Creating relational frames
Countermobilizing	Subgroup threat	Negatively labeling reform practices Denigrating particular reformers Recruiting reformers to defender group
Collectively disrupting	Transient reformers	Interfering with daily activities Pressuring defenders to accommodate a solution that allows them to accomplish their most important goals Legitimating new practices

tural style and status hierarchy. Organization members who claim identities that conflict with traditional roles or who hold marginal positions in the organization are potential internal reformers. Because they are disadvantaged by institutionalized work practices, internal reformers are likely to question existing prescriptions.

Second, the dominant institutionalist approach suggests that the key processes responsible for institutional change happen at the macro level of the organizational field. In this view, change occurs because external reformers disseminate new practices across organizational fields, circulate new compliance programs, create new frames, mobilizing structures, and political opportunities, and fight jurisdictional battles. A micro-institutional focus reveals that to succeed, these change processes, important as they are, must be accompanied by face-to-face collective combat processes occurring on the ground inside organizations.

Third, a traditional institutionalist approach highlights macro-level resources derived from the environment, the organization, or top managers. My approach focuses more on micro-level resources at the small group and face-to-face levels. Defenders and reformers inside similar organizations may be subject to the same environmental pressures and experience the same top-manager support (or opposition) but still act in different ways. Their capacity to collectively resist or press for change is shaped by resources, such as relational spaces, that are available in the particular interactional context in which they are embedded. Table 9.2 highlights the importance of combining macro-level and micro-level explanations.

In sum, the micro-institutional approach I have taken here differs systematically from the macro-institutionalist approach to change. Yet I am not arguing that the macro-institutional approach is wrong. What I am suggesting is that it tells only half the story. For this reason, it is overly simplistic and potentially misleading. We need to understand the other half of the story, the half occurring inside organizations, to fully explain why and how institutional change occurs.

TABLE 9.2. Two levels of institutional change

	MACRO LEVEL	MICRO LEVEL
Primary level of analysis	• Extra-organizational	• Intra-organizational
Focal actors	• Professions • Social movements • Institutional entrepreneurs • Interest groups	• Internal defenders • Diverse subgroups of internal reformers
Institutional change processes	• Advocating professional models • Framing • Building mobilizing structures • Creating political opportunity • Challenging professional jurisdictions	• Defending stability within the organization • Relationally mobilizing within the organization • Countermobilizing within the organization • Collectively disrupting within the organization
Facilitating resources	• Environmental characteristics • Organizational characteristics • Top manager characteristics	• Professional alignment of reformers within the organization • Relational spaces within the organization • Subgroup threat within the organization • Transient reformers within the organization

CONTRIBUTIONS TO FOUR THEORIES OF INSTITUTIONAL CHANGE

Up to this point I have portrayed institutional theory as if it were a homogenous theory whose tenets were universally agreed upon. And I have discussed only the dominant macro-institutionalist approach. But of course there are several different schools of institutional theory, and a handful of theorists within each school have examined micro-level processes of institutional change. Here I look again at four variants of institutional theory—neo-institutional, law and society, social movement, and medical sociology—and note the contributions my study makes to these literatures.

CONTRIBUTIONS TO NEO-INSTITUTIONAL THEORY

Neo-institutionalist theory has established that regulative, normative, and cognitive institutions constrain the behavior of individuals and organizations by distinguishing between legitimate and illegitimate activities.[10] This is borne out by my study. Regulative institutions in surgery required a strict hierarchy with authority, tasks, and responsibilities rigidly prescribed by position. Normative institutions dictated that good residents were Iron Men who were "the first ones there and the last to leave" the hospital. And cognitive institutions suggested that long work hours were required to provide "continuity of care" for patients and "learning by doing" for residents.

However, neo-institutional theorists would not be able to explain who inside hospitals changed the institutionalized practice of handoffs, how they accomplished such a change, and when they were successful in doing so. Regarding *who* accomplishes micro-institutional change, the small group of neo-institutional scholars who have conducted empirical studies inside organizations have demonstrated that low-level actors in addition to top managers are critical for accomplishing change in institutionalized practices.[11] Yet merely including low-level actors does not allow us to explain the difference in outcomes at the hospitals I studied. At Bayshore, low-level actors attempted change. But because they did not build a robust coalition across work positions and social identity groups, they failed to effect it. At Calhoun, low- and mid-level actors did build a coalition but could not sustain it and, in the end, also failed to bring about lasting change. At Advent, low- and mid-level actors created and maintained a coalition, and change occurred.

In explaining *how* institutional change occurs inside organizations, neo-institutional theorists have argued that dominant members in organizations come to embrace new practices favored by marginal members only after marginal members have reinterpreted them in ways the dominant members can understand.[12] But I found that even though reformers at all three hospitals reinterpreted traditional practices, only one reform effort succeeded. In that one instance of success, in the face of fierce resistance, reinterpretation was not enough. This suggests that reformers may be able to get defenders to accommodate new practices only if they also engage in politically charged combat (such as interfering with daily activities, refusing to back down in the face of defender rejection, and ignoring insults). Once such collective disruption has occurred, defenders are more likely to embrace new practices and reinterpret them to address their own goals. They may even use their own high status to help legitimate the new practices—perhaps borrowing some of the frames and identities previously created by reformers.

Finally, regarding the *when* of micro-institutional change, neo-institutional theorists would expect no difference in outcomes across the three hospitals. In their view, change inside organizations stems from external jolts such as shifts in institutional logics or governance structures or from revisions in internal hiring practices that alter the numbers or types of actors brought into organizations.[13] Since the three hospitals I studied were exposed to the same changes in logics and governance structures and since no new kinds of actors were brought into any of them, current theory would predict no variation in institutional change across sites. But I did find variation. Two key factors shaped this variation—differences in availability of relational spaces and differences in the degree of threat posed by the female reformer subgroup. Relational spaces affording isolation from defenders and face-to-face interaction among reformers from multiple work positions were critical to allowing would-be reformers from within Advent and Calhoun to create new tasks, identities, and frames that allowed them to act collectively against defenders of the status quo. Similarly, the weak subgroup threat at Advent allowed male reformers to protect their status in the face of taunts by defenders of the status quo and thus to maintain their male-female reformer coalition long enough to create change.

There are several implications that arise from the discrepancies between my findings and current neo-institutional theory. To explain who is likely to attempt to accomplish institutional change inside organizations, we must examine collective actors inside organizations as well as individual ones. To detail how institutional change occurs inside organizations, we must attend to political processes such as collective disruption in addition to cognitive processes such as reinterpretation and recombination. And to explain when institutional change inside organizations is likely to succeed, we must focus on differences in intra-organizational resources that facilitate reformer coalition building and collective action.

CONTRIBUTIONS TO LAW AND SOCIETY THEORY

The findings of my study contribute to our understanding of how law on the books is prevented from becoming law in action and suggest some implications for law and society theory. Regarding *who* resists change, the general consensus among law and society scholars is that line managers often serve their own material interests by actively discouraging use of the programs established by top managers.[14] At first glance this would seem to be confirmed by my study, for defender residents did pressure interns not to obey the formal rules of the night float program and hand off work to night float members as directors intended. However, upon further reflection, the opposition of the defender residents is surprising since taking on a bit of routine work would seem to be a small price to pay for dramatically reducing their own work hours.

The defender residents at the three hospitals were so strongly alarmed not only because change challenged their material interests but also because it challenged their highly valued codes of appropriate and inappropriate conduct and their customary rationales for traditional practices. When it comes to explaining the behavior of mid-level line managers, law and society theorists undervalue the fact that in addition to material interests, normative and cognitive understandings are important reasons for resistance.[15]

Regarding *how* defenders resisted change, law and society theorists usefully observe how the "naming, blaming, and claiming" game undermines change.[16] Middle managers can prevent subordinates from using programs established by top managers for their benefit by discouraging them from naming a traditional practice as unfair, encouraging them to blame themselves rather than their managers for the perpetuation of traditional practices, and keeping them from claiming their rights for fear of retaliation.[17] Such blocking tactics are powerful and can often dissuade subordinates from using employee rights programs. This was the case when night floats rejected interns' attempts to hand off by claiming that handoff practices were illegitimate, arguing that interns were themselves to blame for needing to work long hours to finish their duties, and drawing on traditional authority relations to persuade interns not to attempt further handoffs.

However, close examination of the "naming, blaming, and claiming" game suggests that it includes a wider variety of tactics than law and society theorists have identified. Defenders at the three hospitals effectively resisted change not only by rejecting handoffs when they were attempted but also by preempting interns' use of the night float program by outlining expectations for how interns should behave, warning them directly about the effects on their reputations if they dared to hand off work, and warning them indirectly by gossiping about interns who did so. Defenders also punished interns who persisted in using the night float programs by loudly and publicly drawing attention to them through "beatings" and by withholding social affiliation and teaching. Further, defenders persuaded one another to take the career risks associating with resisting top manager mandates by building commitment to the defender group and by crafting a set of tactics they could use to resist systematically across situations. Thus, in addition to preventing program use when it is attempted, defenders can block change by preempting attempts to invoke the rights of those who might benefit from a change in the first place, by strongly punishing those who persist, and by organizing with one another.

Finally, regarding *when* institutional change occurs, law and society theorists have noted that when supervisors who administer or authorize participation in a compliance program do not support reform, their subordinates are likely to avoid using the program; conversely, when direct supervisors are supportive, subordinates are likely to feel comfortable invoking their rights.[18] My findings suggest that this may not be entirely true. Interns responded to resistance by ceasing handoff attempts, at least initially, in interactions not only with defender night floats but also with reformer night floats. Since interns were professionals, they cared less about respecting the demands of their direct supervisor than they did about establishing their professional reputation and identity, both of which rested on their acceptance by other professionals (direct supervisors or not) and the training opportunities and career recommendations this could generate.

In sum, there are several discrepancies between my findings and those posited by current law and society theory. To explain who is likely to attempt to resist change in practice in response to regulation, my findings suggest that it is important to attend to the normative identities and cognitive beliefs of mid-level managers in addition to their material interests. To elaborate how compliance is blocked inside organizations, it is important to focus on more than the prevention processes; preemption, punishment, and organizing processes such as those used by defenders in my study are also significant. And to predict when change in daily practice in response to regulation is likely to succeed, it is critical to detail how professional identities and beliefs, in addition to organizational rules and hierarchy, affect compliance.

CONTRIBUTIONS TO SOCIAL MOVEMENT THEORY

My study also suggests implications for theorists interested in how social movements and organizations interact. As these theorists would expect, external patient rights and resident rights reformers created frames and identities, mobilizing structures, and political opportunities for change.[19] Inside all three hospitals, organizational elites who were supportive of work-hours reform—the directors in surgery—developed new policies consistent with reform and committed important resources in the form of night float teams to facilitate reform implementation.[20] Internal reformers were also important to accomplishing work-hours reform, and their access to external and internal resources was related to their success.[21] But regarding *who* the critical players were in shaping outcomes at the three hospitals, internal defenders played as significant a role as did organizational elites and internal reformers. Indeed, internal defenders were key players in undermining the reform attempted within Calhoun.

Regarding *how* reform is accomplished inside organizations, social movement theorists have argued that internal reformers accomplish change using the classic social movement processes used by movements in the streets—they draw on frames, identities, mobilizing structures, and political opportunities provided by external reformers, and they co-opt existing frames, structures, and political opportunities available inside their organizations.[22] However, I found that internal reformers and defenders at the three hospitals attempted and resisted change using a much broader set of change processes. In fact, while actors in all three hospitals engaged in the classic social movement processes of framing, organizing, and creating political opportunity, it was their different levels of engagement in the face-to-face processes of defending stability, relational mobilization, divisive countermobilization, and collective disruption that accounted for the differences in outcomes across the three hospitals.

Finally, regarding *when* reformers were successful in implementing social change, social movement theorists would have expected no difference in outcomes across the three hospitals. Since these theorists believe that successful reform stems from frames, mobilizing structures, and political opportunities available to internal reformers,[23] and since internal reformers at all the hospitals had access to the same set of these resources, social movement theorists would predict that reform would succeed or fail in all three. Yet it succeeded in one and not the other two.

My investigation shows that the actual dynamics were much more complicated. Resources provided by external reformers threatened the professional prestige, authority, and autonomy of the internal reformers, making matters difficult for them. For example, external reformers had framed current practices as unsafe for patients and harmful to residents. As trainees hoping to join the surgical profession, internal reformers had a vested interest in not admitting—as they would have if they had used the same frames as the external reformers—that patient care and their own education had been diminished all along. Thus the interaction-level resources of relational spaces and low subgroup threat ended up being critical to change outcomes in the hospitals—only by using the spaces to create their own new identities and frames and by leveraging the low threat to avoid division in the face of countertactics were internal reformers at Advent able to achieve reform.

The differences between what I found and what current social movement theory would predict suggest that the theory itself needs to be qualified and made more nuanced. To explain who accomplishes reform inside organizations, it is important to examine the role and tactics of internal defenders in addition those of internal reformers. To elaborate how reform implementation occurs, we need to examine the nitty-gritty face-to-face processes that characterize episodes of collective action inside organizations. And to explain when reform implementation is likely to succeed, we must attend to the interaction-level resources that shape mobilization and coalition maintenance.

CONTRIBUTIONS TO MEDICAL SOCIOLOGY

Finally, this book has implications for medical sociologists, who have long been concerned about how, when, and by whom medical practice is controlled. Medical sociologists would not be surprised that the pressure for work-hours reform was brought by a social movement composed of laypeople and experts.[24] Nor would they be surprised that physicians resisted reform, for physicians in the United States have been able to maintain control of their expert knowledge and the high-status position it affords throughout most of the twentieth century by carving out particular task domains and protecting them from competition.[25] The attack on traditional surgical residency practices that I studied was likely particularly threatening to physicians because maintaining control of medical training is a crucial part of protecting professional jurisdiction.[26] As would be expected, medical elites turn to a strategy of self-regulation to protect their jurisdiction.[27] By self-regulating the profession through the ACGME, but then not strictly enforcing work-hours reductions inside hospitals, physicians likely hoped to protect both the profession's control over the field and individual providers' control over routine work activities and decisions.

But what medical sociologists would not be able to account for is who inside hospitals attempted work-hours reform, how they attempted it, and when they were successful in implementing it. Regarding *who* supported reform, the fact that directors in surgery at the three hospitals supported it would have been predicted by medical sociology—the handful of medical sociologists who have conducted ethnographic studies of medical regulation in practice have demonstrated that groups of actors inside hospitals press for reform depending on their professional interests, beliefs, and decision opportunities,[28] and directors had a stake in maintaining the accreditation of their residency programs. But the theory cannot account for why there was variation in support for reform among the residents, even among residents within a particular year of residency. I demonstrate that this variation occurred because reformers within the hospitals were swayed not only by their professional identity and interests as surgeons but also by other salient identities such as woman, husband, or hands-on patient caregiver.

Regarding *how* defenders inside hospitals resisted reform and how reformers attempted it, the few studies that have examined reform implementation have shown that physicians either act individually to resist change (by keeping patients and families on the periphery of decision making) or act individually to support change (by deploying rhetorical strategies to accomplish their goals).[29] Yet I found that both internal defenders and internal reformers acted collectively as well as individually. Defenders shared tactics with one another and built commitment to the defender group to encourage collective resistance; reformers created new relational practices, identities, and frames to encourage collective change.

Finally, medical sociologists trying to explain *when* reformers were successful probably would not have highlighted the key factors that in fact

ended up being important. The few theorists who have examined variation in medical reform implementation across clinical sites describe it as
stemming from differences in the content of reforms (different reforms
afford different costs and benefits to frontline clinicians) and differences in
groups involved across sites (different groups benefit differently from each
reform).[30] Yet both the work-hours reform itself and the mix of providers
involved in implementation was the same at the three hospitals.

What differed across the three hospitals were organizational resources.
Analysis of how variation in resources across organizations shapes different
reform outcomes has been largely absent from medical sociology.[31] My
study shows that directors at all three hospitals offered organizational resources to internal reformers (new accountability systems, staffing systems,
and evaluation systems) that were critical to beginning the reform process.
Further, two key organizational factors were important to creating variation
in outcomes across the hospitals: differences in availability of relational
spaces and differences in the degree of subgroup threat posed by female
reformers.

The discrepancies between my findings and current theory suggest several implications for medical sociology. If we are to predict who is likely
to attempt to accomplish medical reform, it is important to focus on professionals' extra-professional identities and interests, such as those related
to gender or personal life responsibilities, in addition to their professional
identities. To detail how medical reform implementation occurs in day-to-
day work within healthcare settings, it is important to focus on collective
interaction as well as individual interaction. And to explain when reform
implementation is likely to succeed, it is critical to identify how resources
that vary across organizations facilitate change.

RECOMMENDATIONS FOR MEDICAL REFORMERS

At a practical level, my work offers some guidelines to medical reformers.
Arguably, one of the most important challenges facing US medical reformers today is how to implement change in day-to-day practices inside health
care organizations. Over the last few decades, medical costs have risen ex-
ponentially and access to medical care has become a serious problem. Although policies and programs to address these issues have proliferated, they
have not dramatically changed day-to-day work practices.[32] We should not
be surprised at all by this failure to transform daily medical practices. Implementing reform often means challenging long-standing medical institu-

tions. However, as I have shown, though implementation may be difficult, it is not impossible.

As we have seen in the case of resident work-hours reform, political opportunities, mobilizing structures, frames, and identities useful to those outside and inside healthcare organizations are likely to be different. Thus, as a practical matter, external reformers in health care should consider developing two sets of resources: one for the general public and medical reformer elites and another for internal reformers.

First, political opportunities helpful to medical elites are those like the eighty-hour workweek regulation that pressure medical administrators to be more accountable to outside regulators. However, such political opportunities, while critical for change, may be less helpful to internal reformers. Indeed, none of the reformers I observed reported work-hours violations to the ACGME even though they were aware that violations were occurring. To make the political opportunity of new regulation helpful to internal reformers, social movements should press for strong whistleblower protection and for national legislation rather than medical self-regulation. In the case of work-hours reform, external reformers have been savvy enough to do both but have met with mixed success to date. AMSA has argued for whistleblower protection using the case of Troy Madsen, a resident who was disgraced among his colleagues after he informed the ACGME of work-hours violations at Johns Hopkins Hospital. After Madsen's whistleblowing came to light, the work environment became so hostile that he felt he had little choice but to transfer to a residency program at Ohio State University. Social movement reformers have publicized the Madsen case, and in its 2008 review the IOM responded to their pressure by recommending that the ACGME create more robust whistleblower protections and find alternative procedures that would shield the identity of whistleblowers when they report violations.[33]

Work-hours reformers have also pressed for national rather than professional regulation, using anonymous surveys and anecdotal accounts to argue that work hours are systematically misreported across many programs. Organizations like AMSA have underwritten studies, conducted anonymous surveys, and provided web and print forums for residents to make their stories heard while protecting anonymity. The IOM reviewed this information in its 2008 report and has recommended that the Centers for Medicare and Medicaid Services begin to assess the reliability of ACGME procedures and data and periodically provide independent reviews of ACGME's monitoring (but that the profession remain responsible for regulating work hours).[34] The evidence presented in this book suggests that these IOM recommendations are important but may not go far enough for broad reform implementation to occur; airtight whistleblower protection is critical, and national regulation could provide internal reformers with stronger political opportunities for challenge within their hospitals than will better supervised self-regulation.

Second, organizations and networks such as the reform conferences that have been held by work-hours reformers may be of great assistance to reform-minded medical elites in helping them identify problems, evaluate solutions, learn of new tactics, and create a collective sense of agency and solidarity. But these mobilizing structures may not be as useful to reformers inside healthcare organizations, who are likely to be quite concerned about how fraternizing with public crusaders would negatively affect their career. Since internal reformers cannot join with external reformers without risking their reputation within the profession, external reformers should consider holding separate forums devoted to organizing internal reformers.

Finally, the frames and identities that help external reformers and reform-minded medical elites to raise public opposition to accepted healthcare practices are likely to be those (such as the Libby Zion case) that dramatize glaring deficiencies in these practices. Yet while frames and identities that paint current medical practices as unsafe for patients may be useful for prodding the general public into action, they are not useful to reformers on the front lines inside hospitals, many of whom are reluctant to change everyday practices at the cost of undermining their own professional status. Thus external reformers should consider fashioning specific frames for internal reformers.[35] In the case of work-hours reform, social movements might develop an oppositional consciousness in male internal reformers with personal life responsibilities by narrowing their frames to target just this, emphasizing for instance the specific difficulties male surgical residents face in juggling work and family and thus perhaps motivating men in this group to become more politically active.[36]

External reformers should also consider more sophisticated ways of dealing with issues of identity. Since most defenders belong to higher-status social categories, they are able to devalue the reformer identity by singling out particular lower-status reformer subgroups. In the case of work-hours reform, Iron Men deprecated male reformers by assigning them feminine labels. To encourage higher-status internal reformers to engage in collective action to improve their group's status rather than defecting to the higher-status defender group, external reformers may need to emphasize the impermeability of the defender group boundary by challenging defender claims about the openness of their group. In the case of work-hours reform, social movements could raise consciousness by showing how empty was the promise that residents could "trust no one" and still deliver complex, team-based care.

RECOMMENDATIONS FOR MEDICAL ADMINISTRATORS

While social movements can provide general resources to reformers from the outside, medical administrators can provide organization-specific resources to them from the inside. The findings presented here suggest that administrators can facilitate reform by using reformer-friendly accountability, staffing, and evaluation systems. In addition, medical administrators can encourage change by attending to issues of gender and hierarchy when implementing new programs.

Reformer-friendly programs such as new accountability systems can make middle managers responsible for change and thereby legitimate open support for reform. Until the directors at Advent, Bayshore, and Calhoun assigned the chief residents accountability for change, I observed few chiefs who were willing to agitate overtly for change. But once the directors made chief residents accountable, reformers who had earlier kept silent about their beliefs began to openly support change. They felt emboldened to do so because the new accountability system meant that they would be supported in their actions by top managers.[37]

Medical administrators can also offer internal reformers new staffing systems that allow them to coordinate their efforts with one another. In the cases presented here, the absence of a new staffing system before the beginning of the new resident year meant that there was no opportunity for reformers from different work positions to coordinate their efforts. But once the new night float teams were put into place, reformers were able to work together to create a set of supporting practices that led to reform. My findings suggest that a particular type of staffing system is most helpful—one that allows reformers to work and mobilize together in the absence of defenders. Those who support change must have their own meeting spaces that allow supporters across different work positions to build a committed group for change. Such spaces play an especially critical role because supporters of change are often uncomfortable trying out new tasks, playing new roles, or discussing nontraditional ideas when defenders of the status quo are present.

Another way healthcare administrators can help reformers is to provide them with nonrepressive evaluation systems that will allow them to collectively challenge defenders. In the cases presented here, the absence of new evaluation systems before the beginning of the new resident year meant that quite often reformers were punished for attempting change. As a result, they came to fear the consequences of collective challenge. To the degree they contested traditional practices, they did so in acts of resistance that were individual and covert. Directors at the three hospitals ameliorated reformers' fears when they began to informally ask how the new night float team was working and urge chiefs to name any night floats who were refusing to take handoffs of scutwork from the interns. The informal discussion put into place by this new evaluation system was critical, because the only other way for chiefs to tell directors about defender resistance was formal notification, and that would have required residents to violate the professional norm of "covering each other's back."

Gender and hierarchy also have important roles to play in the implementation of new programs. For example, the IOM's key recommendation is the introduction of a protected sleep period of five hours during any work shift of more than sixteen hours. Yet the IOM committee itself acknowledges that "while a protected nighttime sleep of up to 4–5 hours duration appears feasible as a way to prevent acute sleep deprivation in resident physicians during an extended duty period, the limited data available indicate that adherence to such a schedule was relatively poor (22–56 percent)."[38] The report goes on to say that "resident unwillingness to obtain sleep when a protected period with pager handoff to others is available appears to be due to their concerns about the patients they admitted, continuity of care, and their own workload."[39] Because the IOM diagnoses poor adherence to a program of protected nighttime sleep as an issue of concern over continuity of care, one of the solutions it recommends is "using more experienced physicians to cover patients for them so residents will have less cause for concern about their patients."[40]

The idea that adherence to protected sleep could be improved by requiring residents to hand off their work to senior physicians is simply ludicrous in surgical residency given its strongly hierarchical structure. In addition, the new requirement of a nap will face serious challenge in the macho culture of surgical residency.

Yet the scientific evidence clearly shows that preventing acute sleep loss in residents is critical to patient safety. So what is a reformer administrator to do in the face of the new nap requirement? Let me suggest two courses of action. First, administrators should minimize subgroup threat in the organization by studiously avoiding the creation of any visible programs for female residents that appear to favor females as a group.[41] In the absence of a subgroup threat, defenders will have a harder time devaluing male reformers who use the new protected sleep program. Second, administrators should structure the program so that residents of the same level or lower (rather than more senior residents or attendings) are covering the resident's work during protected sleep periods.

RECOMMENDATIONS FOR MEDICAL PROVIDERS

While medical administrators can provide resources to internal reformers, frontline medical providers inside healthcare organizations are critical to fighting for change in everyday organizational practices in ways that others cannot. The findings presented in this book suggest that internal reformers can most effectively accomplish change by thinking collectively, identifying other potential reformers, seeking out relational spaces, minimizing the threat of reformer subgroups, and enlisting transients. Although the necessity of collective action for change is patently obvious to social movement theorists, it is not the first thing to spring to the minds of those inside organizations when they attempt reform. This seems particularly true for high-status professionals. At the three hospitals I studied, residents who wanted to implement work-hours reduction did not think about how they could engage others in the cause. They attempted to use or support the new night float programs, but they did so as individuals, not as a collective group. As a consequence, they were summarily defeated (at least initially) by defenders of the status quo.

Internal reformers too often see their problems as theirs alone. They may feel guilty about attempting change because close friends embrace the status quo. They may worry that acting collectively will lead people to brand them as reformers and judge them negatively. It is safer, they think, to resist quietly and individually. But when powerful defenders of the status quo fiercely resist change, individual change attempts fail. The force of valued roles, long-standing authority relations, and traditional narratives is simply too great for would-be reformers to individually overcome.

To identify others who share their goals, then, is a challenge for internal reformers. They are not always aware of one another. At the three hospitals studied here, reformers initially had no idea that many others shared their cause and goals. Organization members who question traditional practices often do not voice their support for reform. Would-be internal reformers, however, can gauge how much others are likely to support change by noting their social identities. Organizational members with identities that are disadvantaged in society-at-large often receive fewer rewards and opportunities for training and promotion inside organizations than do their counterparts.[42] They are more likely than others to be potential reformers.

Since shared communication settings have been shown to reduce conflict, one might think that those who seek change would do well to bring defenders and reformers together to plan and implement compliance programs jointly. However, my study suggests the opposite. Instead, in organizing their efforts, reformers must find spaces that provide isolation from defenders. Such spaces are critical because reformers are not comfortable talking about and trying out new ways to do things when defenders are present. Interaction apart from work itself is also crucial because it facilitates time for discussing new ways of working. And inclusion of reformers from all the work positions involved in the practice targeted for change is important because it enables collective coordination and negotiation.

Finally, coalitions composed of numerous subgroups are only as strong as their weakest link, it seems, and keeping this link out of the limelight may be a tactic of considerable worth. For example, female managers in a male-dominated organization who choose to dine as a group may do best to hide this from their male colleagues. In addition, activism requires significant effort and risks the loss of important rewards. One might imagine, therefore, that those most committed to a cause will be the most significant reformers. But I have suggested that those moving through organizations— the less committed transients—may be, in the end, the most effective change agents. They have less at stake and worry less about their reputation, for they will soon be gone. Thus they may be willing to engage in the most direct challenge to defenders and can be critical fighters in the change effort if the change benefits them immediately.

A FINAL WORD

At the broadest level, I have tried to demonstrate that institutional change at the macro level does not automatically translate into institutional change on the ground inside organizations. Institutional entrepreneurs, professional groups, social movements, and interest groups outside of workplaces may fight for new regulations designed to produce social change inside. But without internal reformers engaging in collective combat against defenders of the status quo, institutional change is not likely to occur.

Why don't regulations act as unilateral directives that force organizations to change? They don't because organizations often adopt new policies or programs to create believable displays of conformity for external audiences but then decouple formal policies and programs from actual daily practices. Depending on one's view of change, this may or may not be a problem. In some cases, new regulations are designed by outsiders who do not understand how to best require or measure change. In other cases, regulations do not address the organizational issues that all members believe need attention. But even when new regulations are well designed and address issues that will help level the playing field for disadvantaged organization members or customers, they are often resisted by powerful internal defenders of the status quo.

The key argument of this book is that organization members who would benefit from institutional change (and their supporters) must understand how to effectively engage in face-to-face collective combat processes if they are to successfully accomplish it. To bring to fruition the opportunities hard won by external reformers, reformers inside organizations must successfully find relational spaces apart from defenders of the status quo to coordinate their efforts across diverse work positions and social identities. They must stand up to aggressive attempts to divide their coalition. And they must enlist transient reformers to put their necks on the line for the cause. Only by engaging in such tenacious collective combat can internal reformers accomplish the institutional change that those outside have fought so hard to promote.

Acknowledgments

I am deeply indebted to the people whose wonderful ideas and support made this book possible.

Lotte Bailyn has been an incredible source of inspiration, and my relationship with her has truly been life-changing. Her research on work–personal life integration as a societal rather than personal problem and on collective action for change has made me look at the world in a new way. She continues to challenge me to question the status quo, envision how things could be different, and write about what I am finding.

John Van Maanen has taught me the craft of ethnography and the approach of the Chicago School. At his urging I have tried to get as close to my informants as possible, to become a "Convert" rather than a "Martian," to draw a broad cultural portrait from focusing on everyday happenings, to provide detail on these day-to-day situations, and to get rid of my 300,000-feet variables (I tried, John, I swear I tried). John has provided line-by-line feedback to help me better tell the story.

It was Wanda Orlikowski who introduced me to the incredibly liberating idea that we construct the world we live in and we have the responsibility and challenge to "act otherwise." Wanda has helped me find my academic voice and encouraged me to use it. Leslie Perlow has taught me to "trust the method." Her constant refrain of "What's the story really about?" has pushed me to go back to the data again and again in search of insights, and her confident "If it is really important, it will happen again" was critical to my peace of mind during fieldwork. I am also grateful to Roberto Fernandez, who has challenged me to be a "column person as well as a row person" and to figure out which theoretical conversations I want to enter. His feedback has encouraged me to solve puzzles rather than fill gaps in the literature, to sharpen the connection between my processes and outcomes, and to use my stories to contribute to theory. Ezra Zuckerman has led me to "frame around the dependent variable," to start with the question rather than with my answer to it. His suggestions about building up the interesting alternatives to my argument have been critical to my thinking.

My warmest thanks to others who helped: to the Alfred P. Sloan Foundation for generous financial support; to Doug Mitchell and Tim McGovern at the University of Chicago Press for believing in and guiding this book; to two anonymous reviewers who provided careful and insightful feedback; to Bill Gamson for introducing me to social movements and the micro-mechanisms associated with them; to Doug McAdam for leading me to redraft the conclusions for greater theoretical impact; to Dick Scott for enthusiastically encouraging me to tell more of the macro-level story; to Mayer Zald for helping me hone my countermobilization analysis; to Frank Dobbin for making connections between my work and law and society theory; to Cal Morrill for thoughts on the relationship between organization structure and defender resistance; to Carol Heimer for leading me to engage with medical sociology; to Steve Barley for mentorship on ethnography and the "coalface"; to Maureen Scully and Debra Meyerson for feedback on micro-institutional change; to Woody Powell for the idea of making relational spaces more concrete; to Huggy Rao for encouraging me to report comparative findings; to Rick Locke and Lucio Baccaro for guidance on the craft of comparative case study research; to Susan Silbey for highlighting the interplay between culture and power; to Mauro Guillen, Paul Osterman, Michel Anteby, and Victoria Johnson for advice on book writing; to JoAnne Yates for thoughts on historical analysis; to Deborah Ancona for help on academic identity; to John Carroll for insights into patient safety; to Tom Kochan for inspiring me to solve real-world problems; to Ray Reagans for ideas about subgroup visibility and resistance; to Jesper Sorensen for urging me to tell less rather than more, but coherently; to Ann Bookman, Pablo Boczkowski, and Paul Carlile for helping with fieldwork challenges; to Mabel Abraham, Sujata Bhat, Casey Brock-Wilson, and Ryan Hammond for research assistance; to Barbara Feinman, Dennis Todd, and Ruth Goring for excellent editorial help; to Megan Wilkins for great administrative assistance; to the MIT Economic Sociology Working Group for talk about framing, the HBS QUIET group for talk about ethnographic methods, the KVEJJ group for talk about careers, and the Boston College MRAP group for talk about social change; to my faculty friends Sarah Kaplan and Isabel Fernandez for sharp insights at multiple stages and Corinne Bendersky, Forrest Briscoe, Rodrigo Canales, Emilio Castilla, Lisa Cohen, Sachi Hatakenaka, Denise Lewin-Loyd, Melissa Mazmanian, Mark Mortensen, Yiorgos Mylonadis, Brian Rubineau, Lourdes Sosa, Sean Safford, and Chris Wheat for great feedback on related work; to my college friends Cynthia Braun for medical editing and Pam Codispoti, Tricia Grant, Sarah Jackson-Han, and Jane Lonnquist for hearing more about the Iron Man over the years than anyone should ever have to know; to Kate Dempsey for wonderful caregiving help; to Lois Slovik for reinforcing why it's great for kids to have two working parents; to Jane Brock-Wilson for career bullishness; to Katelyn Quynn for being my fellow working mother of boys; and to Leslie Tsui for weekly walks around the pond.

As an ethnographer, I aim to describe the world of surgical residents from the perspective of those who live it. I also need to make sure to protect all of the people who so generously gave me their time and their insights from any unwanted ramifications from my research. For this reason, I have used pseudonyms for the individuals I studied, and this precludes me from publicly thanking the people who took me into their confidence and shared their experiences and their hopes for the future with me. But those whose lives are depicted in this book know who they are, and to them I am deeply indebted. Thank you for putting up with my endless barrage of questions, and for always greeting me with a smile when I showed up with my notepad for yet another day of following you around. You will likely never know how much you affected me or how much I learned from you. I hope that I have done justice to your experiences and the complexity of your world.

My family has been tremendously supportive of my work. My brother Jimmy Kellogg and sister Elizabeth Winterbottom have smiled indulgently at my academic approach to life and helped with pragmatic advice when needed. My mother- and father-in-law Catherine and Don Peeler, my aunt and uncle Betsy and Rusty Kellogg, and my parents Gail and Jim Kellogg have provided much-needed reinforcement at all of my pressure points. My mom's morning cell phone calls and "you can do it" attitude were terrifically helpful. My dad has read many drafts of the work and provided great comments at each step: "It's actually a lot more interesting to read than most academic books," he's assured me. My boys, Chris and Andrew, have been huge fans of Professor/Mom, made several illustrated versions of the promised book, and given me hugs and laughter every day. Randy Peeler, my partner on this journey, has been more important to me than I can say. He has been a believer from the beginning, an unwavering reader, a fantastic father, and a wonderful husband.

Thank you.

Notes

PREFACE

1. Bailyn 2006 [1993].

INTRODUCTION

1. Quoted in Garrett 1995.
2. Perez-Pena 1994.
3. For a description of the grand jury conclusions, see New York Supreme Court 1986. In 1995, further court proceedings about Zion's death raised questions about whether duty hours and supervision were the only contributing factors; assigning blame was complicated because when she was admitted to the hospital Zion did not report the conflicting medicines she was taking (Andrews 1995; Douglas 1995).
4. McCall 1988, 776–78.
5. New York State Department of Health 1989.
6. Drummond et al. 2000; Harrison and Horne 2000; Kleitman 1963; Patrick and Gilbert 1896; Portas et al. 1998; Thomas et al. 2000.
7. Friedman, Bigger, and Kornfield 1971.
8. Grantcharov et al. 2001.
9. Gaba and Howard 2002; Pilcher and Huffcutt 1996; Samkoff and Jacques 1991; Veasey et al. 2002; Weinger and Ancoli-Israel 2002.
10. Boodman 2001.
11. Kowalenko et al. 2000; Marcus and Loughlin 1996; Parks et al. 2000; Steele et al. 1999.

12. Grunebaum, Minkoff, and Blake 1987; Klebanoff, Shiono, and Rhoads 1990; Pitts et al. 1979; Reuben 1985; Valko and Clayton 1975.
13. Rubinowitz 1999.
14. Public Citizen 2001.
15. HR 3236 2001.
16. Laine et al. 1993.
17. Petersen et al. 1994.
18. Steinbrook 2002.
19. Ibid.
20. Landrigan et al. 2004.
21. IOM 2008, 6.
22. ACGME 2004.
23. *New York Times* 2008.
24. Barnard 2002.
25. Bell 2003, 37.
26. *New York Times* 2002, cited in Bell 2003, 37.
27. Steinbrook 2002.
28. Chang 2004.
29. Strazouso 2004.
30. Zeigler 2005.
31. Landrigan et al. 2006.
32. DiMaggio and Powell 1983; Edelman 1992; Meyer and Rowan 1977; Oliver 1991; Silbey 1981.
33. DiMaggio 1991b; Fligstein 1997; Greenwood et al. 2008; Powell 1991; Scott 2007; Tolbert and Zucker 1996.
34. DiMaggio 1988; Hardy and Maguire 2008.
35. Haveman and Rao 1997; Powell 1991.
36. John Sutton and Frank Dobbin (1996) demonstrate how central actors help innovations become accepted once they are introduced by institutional entrepreneurs. But also see Greenwood and Suddaby 2006 for an explanation of how change is sometimes initiated from the center of mature organizational fields.
37. Hinings et al. 2004.
38. DiMaggio 1991a; Greenwood, Suddaby, and Hinings 2002.
39. Fligstein 1997; Suchman 1995.
40. Baron, Dobbin, and Jennings 1986; Edelman, Uggen, and Erlanger 1999; Guillén 1994; Tolbert and Zucker 1983.
41. Oliver 1992.
42. Fox-Wolfgramm, Boal, and Hunt 1998; Mezias and Scarselletta 1994; Palmer, Jennings, and Zhou 1993.
43. Alexander 1996; Fligstein 1985; Rao, Monin, and Durand 2005.
44. Dobbin 2009; Edelman and Stryker 2005; Edelman and Suchman 1997; Heimer 1996; Kelly 2010; Kelly and Kalev 2006; Morrill 1995; Silbey, Huising, and Coslovsky 2009; Suchman and Edelman 2007.
45. Kelly 2003; Silbey 1981; Sutton and Dobbin 1996.
46. Edelman, Abraham, and Erlanger 1992; Edelman et al. 1991.
47. Dobbin 2009; Dobbin and Kelly 2007; Dobbin et al. 1993; Edelman, Uggen,

and Erlanger 1999; Kalev and Dobbin 2006; Kelly and Dobbin 1999; Sutton, et al. 1994.
48. Edelman 1990; Edelman 1992; Morrill 1998; Sutton et al. 1994.
49. Dobbin et al. 1993; Edelman, Fuller, and Mara-Drita 2001; Kelly and Dobbin 1998.
50. Edelman 1990; Edelman 1992; Kalev, Shenhav, and De Vries 2008; Silbey 1981.
51. Baron, Dobbin, and Jennings 1986; Dobbin et al. 1988; Edelman, Abraham, and Erlanger 1992; Mezias 1990.
52. Edelman et al. 1991; Heimer 1999; Silbey, Huising, and Coslovsky 2009.
53. Clemens 2005; Davis et al. 2005; Davis et al. 2008; Haveman, Rao, and Paruchuri 2007; Lounsbury, Ventresca, and Hirsch, 2003; McAdam and Scott 2005; Morrill, Zald, and Rao 2003; Rao, Morrill, and Zald 2000; Soule 2009; Zald 2008; Zald, Morrill, and Rao 2005.
54. McAdam and Scott 2005.
55. Gamson 1992a; McAdam, McCarthy, and Zald 1996; Rao, Monin, and Durand 2003; Snow et al. 1986; Taylor and Whittier 1992.
56. McCann 1994.
57. Clemens 1993; McCarthy and Zald 1977.
58. King 2008; King and Soule 2007; McAdam 1999 [1982]; Soule 2009.
59. In addition to external resources, internal resources such as networks or task forces that reformers can use to mobilize together are critical for reform implementation (e.g., Meyerson 2003 [2001]; Raeburn 2004).
60. Creed and Scully 2000; Creed, Scully, and Austin 2002.
61. Moore 2008; Raeburn 2004.
62. Binder 2002; Katzenstein 1998.
63. Katzenstein 1998; Taylor and Raeburn 1995; Zald, Morrill, and Rao 2005.
64. Morrill, Zald, and Rao 2003; Zald, Morrill, and Rao 2005.
65. Abbott 1988; Bird et al. 2010; Brown and Zavestoski 2005; Conrad 2008; Freidson 1986; Hafferty and Light 1995; Light 2000; Quadagno 2004; Starr 1982.
66. Banaszak-Holl, et al. 2010; Light 2000; Taylor and Zald 2010; Taylor 1996.
67. McAdam and Scott 2005; Scott et al. 2000.
68. Conrad and Schneider 1992; Freidson 1986; Larson 1977; Starr 1982.
69. Zetka 2003.
70. Fox 1959; Galison and Stump 1996.
71. McAdam and Scott 2005; Scott et al. 2000; Taylor and Zald 2010.
72. For example, Stefan Timmermans and Marc Berg (2003) have argued that the movement toward evidence-based medicine can be seen as physicians' attempt to regain the public's trust and safeguard the profession's status by emphasizing the scientific foundation of their work.
73. Ibid.
74. Anspach 1993; Bosk 1992; Chambliss 1996; Heimer and Staffen 1998; Timmermans and Berg 2003; Zussman 1992. This ethnographic research provides a more micro-level view of the control over medical work than much of the research described in this introduction, and I will revisit it in more detail in my conclusions.

75. Heimer 1999; Timmermans and Berg 2003.
76. Conrad 2008.
77. For a description of the ethnographic method, see Van Maanen 1988.
78. Thanks to John Van Maanen for this excellent advice.
79. On ethnographic interviewing, see Spradley 1979.
80. Forty-three directors, attendings, chiefs, seniors, and interns were interviewed at both points. An additional seven residents were interviewed only once.
81. Glaser and Strauss 1967.

CHAPTER 1

1. To protect the confidentiality of my informants and the hospitals in which they worked, all names are pseudonyms. All events occurred as reported, and pseudonyms have been chosen with attention to important characteristics such as the gender and ethnicity of the real people involved. Characteristics unimportant to the analysis, such as the residents' hair color, number of children, or hometown, the hospitals' general surgery floor numbers, and the city's hotel names have been altered to protect confidentiality.
2. In this chapter I purposely do not indicate at which hospital these observations were made. Residents at the three hospitals worked similar hours doing similar things before the regulation.
3. While this comment was directed toward nurses, I never saw a doctor alphabetize these notebooks either.
4. Terry Mizrahi (1986) argues that one of the key things residents learn during residency is how to get rid of patients. She describes how they do this by transferring patients to another service or to a more junior resident. However, Charles Bosk (2003 [1979]) has pointed out that in addition to learning how to get through the day by avoiding as much scutwork as possible, residents also learn to take responsibility for issues that are critical to patient care, even when that involves deferring their own needs.
5. Robert Zussman (1992) makes a similar point about intellectually interesting cases in his book on adult ICUs. Competitive banter can also be seen as what Michel Anteby (2008) refers to as an "identity incentive."
6. Association of American Medical Colleges 2009; US Bureau of Labor Statistics 2002.
7. It was actually rare for residents to comment on my outsider status when I was observing them. I think Anne did so here because I had followed her for such an extended period. The demands of the residents' work were so great and so urgent that I was a relatively unimportant person in their social world. They grew accustomed to me, and I felt that my presence did not affect the change process in any significant way, if at all.
8. As noted in the introduction, I do not have hard indicators of the negative consequences of the long hours for these three hospitals. The absence of negative consequence data is an important matter, but it reflects the ACGME and hospitals' measurement systems rather than my own omission. Since there are many care providers involved in surgical patient care,

there are too many confounding effects to be able to measure this without a controlled study of medical errors that closely tracks all these inputs in addition to resident work hours and errors. As I will discuss in my concluding chapter, such studies are critical to measuring the effect of reduced work hours on patients and residents themselves. However, while measurements are valuable and necessary, they don't tell the whole story. The ethnographic study presented in this book is extremely well suited to telling a different part of this story—how and why work-hours change occurred (or not) on the ground inside of hospitals.

CHAPTER 2

1. Law and society theorists have demonstrated that, to be effective, regulation requires clear demands, adequate surveillance, and significant sanctions (e.g. Baron, Dobbin, and Jennings 1986; Edelman 1990).
2. Zeigler 2004.
3. Bell 2003.
4. Kennedy 1998.
5. Social movement theorists suggest that several factors are important to the emergence of a movement: frames, identities, mobilizing structures, and political opportunities. Frames are action-oriented sets of beliefs and meanings that diagnose conditions as problems and offer corrective prognoses to motivate collective action (e.g., Gamson 1988; Snow and Benford 1988). Frames also provide identities of protagonists and antagonists by distinguishing "us" from "them" and suggesting specifiable lines of actions for contenders (e.g.. Gamson 1988; Hunt, Benford, and Snow 1994; Jasper and Polletta 2001). Mobilizing structures are informal and formal collective vehicles, such as groups, organizations, and networks, through which people can mobilize and engage in collective action (e.g. McCarthy and Zald 1977). And political opportunities are changes in the institutional structure or informal power relations of a political system that make the system more vulnerable or receptive to the demands of particular groups (McAdam 1999 [1982]).
6. Social movement theorists have argued that particular environmental conditions such as elite disunity make the existing system vulnerable to challenge and therefore present "political opportunities" for reformers (McAdam 1999 [1982]; Tarrow 1994).
7. Zinner 2002.
8. A physician compensation and production survey of medical professionals showed that in 2004 general surgeons made an average salary of $278,000. The Bureau of Labor Statistics (US Bureau of Labor Statistics 2002) reports that the 2002 mean pay for surgeons in the United States was $190,000. While private compensation reports reflect a much higher salary, the BLS survey allows for a comparison of surgeon salaries to those of other professionals. At the BLS estimate of $190,000, surgeons were paid significantly more than social workers ($39,000), reporters ($39,000), clergy ($36,000), teachers ($44,000), scientists ($66,000), architects ($63,000),

computer software engineers ($76,000), judges ($85,000), and lawyers ($106,000). In addition to being paid more than non-physicians, US surgeons were paid more than US doctors in other medical specialties. The Physician Compensation and Production Survey (Medical Group Management Association 2009) showed that in 2004 general surgeons made an average salary of $278,000 compared to $216,000 for emergency medicine doctors, $166,000 for internal medicine doctors, and $152,000 for family practitioners. Finally, surgeons in the United States were among the highest paid in the developed world. A survey of specialists in the United States versus other OECD countries conducted by the US Congressional Research Service (2007) showed that, adjusted for purchasing power parity, US specialists, with an average salary of $230,000 earned more than specialists in all other developed countries except the Netherlands and Australia; the median salary for specialists in all OECD countries was $83,000. To be fair, these numbers do not take into account the fact that doctors in other OECD countries pay much less for their medical education than do their US counterparts and so start their medical careers with much less debt.

9. Harris Interactive 2009.
10. Dunn and Miller 1997; Rosoff and Leone 1991.
11. Freidson 1988.
12. John McKinlay and Lisa Marceau (2002) describe the loss of the golden age of doctoring. Attendings and residents told me that the loss of patient trust was reflected in the rise in medical malpractice premiums. But Tom Baker (2007) concludes that the real problem is too much medical malpractice (actual errors), not too much litigation. He finds that since people frequently do not sue, it is the victims rather than doctors who bear the real costs of medical malpractice.
13. For a historical analysis of radiology's inroads into surgical jurisdictions, see Zetka 2003.
14. Zinner 2002.
15. Neumayer et al. 2002.
16. The ACGME evaluates each residency program every three to four years with site visits and resident interviews to examine the content of training and ensure compliance with ACGME requirements.
17. Neo-institutional theorists have highlighted a set of specific organizational characteristics that have been shown to explain variation in change outcomes in response to external pressure. Differences in organization size and alignment with the public sector promote variation because some regulative requirements apply only to organizations of a given size and because larger organizations are more visible to external constituencies (Edelman 1992; Greening and Gray 1994; Mezias 1990). Differences in organizational performance history and image promote variation because organizations with poor performance histories have been shown to decouple formal programs from daily practices and because organizations have been shown to resist change attempts that are inconsistent with their identity and image (Fox-Wolfgramm, Boal, and Hunt 1998; Westphal and Zajac 1994).
18. Edelman 1992; Greening and Gray 1994; Mezias 1990.

19. Davis and Greve 1997; Palmer, Jennings, and Zhou 1993.
20. Fox-Wolfgramm, Boal, and Hunt 1998.
21. For a discussion of middle-status conformity, see Phillips and Zuckerman 2001.
22. Westphal and Zajac 1994.
23. Alexander 1996; Fligstein 1985; Rao, Monin, and Durand 2005.
24. Raeburn 2004; Scully and Segal 2002; Strang and Jung 2005.
25. The New York experience had not proved that night float teams were the most effective way to reduce surgical resident work hours. In fact, New York hospitals had used a mix of overlapping strategies on top of night float teams: increasing the responsibilities of existing PAs (physician assistants), NPs (nurse practitioners), and ancillary staff (e.g., phlebotomists or EKG technicians); adding new staff in these areas; increasing the cross-coverage of patients; shifting duties from junior to senior residents; allowing residents to take call from home; and recruiting new residents (Whang et al. 2003). While introducing night float teams was the most common staffing model used by New York hospitals to comply with the new regulation, no single approach to staffing had been definitively shown to be effective. Edward Whang et al. (2003) show that in addition to introducing night float teams (50 percent), two other strategies were used frequently by New York academic medical centers: increasing cross-coverage of patients (57 percent) and increasing the responsibilities of PAs and NPs or adding new ones (58 percent). Because these two strategies primarily involve shifting work around within the current team, I do not refer to them as new staffing models.

    We should not be surprised that directors at the three hospitals turned to New York for guidance when it came time to develop new programs. Often a model adopted early, like the night float team model, proven or not, can later have a significant impact on the field as a whole. Institutional theorists have demonstrated that organizations responding first to a new regulation (such as hospitals in New York State) frequently try to craft a model that regulators would likely see as legitimate, and organizations that respond later (such as hospitals in other areas of the country) are likely to copy models that appear to have succeeded, instead of creating new models that might be more efficient for them (Edelman 1992; Sutton et al. 1994).
26. IOM 2008.

CHAPTER 3

1. Institutional theorists have shown how people inside organizations, rather than acting rationally to maximize their material interests are embedded in a web of cultural, political, and cognitive understandings—institutions— that shape their actions as well those of others in the social system (DiMaggio 1991b; Meyer and Rowan 1977; Scott 2007). Medical sociologists have explained how doctors learn these cultural, political, and cognitive understandings as part of their medical training. For foundational work in this area, see Becker 1961; Bosk 2003 [1979]; Fox 1957; Hughes 1971; Merton,

Reader, and Kindall 1957. For more recent work, see Brosnan and Turner 2009.

2. Cassell 1998.

3. Katz 1999.

4. Bosk 2003 [1979].

5. Siddhartha Mukherjee (2002) discusses the history of Halsted's system. Harvard sleep researcher Charles Czeisler (2009) points out that Halsted himself had a cocaine addiction, which may have perhaps clouded his judgment as to how many hours physicians could safely work.

6. This high position in the professional hierarchy has also been sustained by restrictions on the supply of surgeons. In his historical analysis of intraprofessional competition between surgeons and gastroenterologists, James Zetka (2003) details how the surgical profession has fought to protect its jurisdiction by limiting the number of surgical residency positions.

7. Culture researchers have demonstrated how cultural tools such as roles, positional understandings, and legitimating accounts provide a "toolkit" of resources that organization members can use to develop and shape strategies of action in particular situations as they go about their day-to-day work (Fine 1996; Swidler 2001; Vaughan 1996).

8. Blackbourne 1996, 4.

9. Andrew Abbott (1988, 118–19), discusses how frontline client service work such as this has lower status than academic work and so is often relegated to low-status professional colleagues such as residents.

10. Erving Goffman (1956) and William Whyte (1949) explain how underlings reinforce their status with one another by attending to minute deference behaviors.

11. Bucher and Stelling 1977; Conrad 1988; Light 1980.

12. Becker 1960; Becker 1961; Carper and Becker 1957.

13. Despite this strong belief, research has shown that continuity of care, even in the traditional system, was experienced by a small percentage of surgical residents (Anderson et al. 1996).

14. The rationale of "learning by doing" is not unique to surgery. It is much the same as the rationales described by scholars studying other occupations where craft is necessary. In craft-centered occupations, physical or manual talent is considered critical. Sense of materials and situations is seen as being essential to performance, because the kinds of problems artisans typically face often require them to solve problems immediately with whatever materials they have at hand (e.g., Barley 1996).

15. Mukherjee 2004, 1824,.

16. Roger Friedland and Robert Alford (1991), Elisabeth Clemens and James Cook (1999), and Myeong-gu Seo and Douglas Creed (2002) have theorized about how actors can exploit internal contradictions to create space for institutional change. Carol Heimer (1999) and Thomas D'Aunno, Melissa Succi, and Jeffrey Alexander (2000) have shown how actors inside of hospitals draw on competing institutions to make decisions about patient care. And Calvin Morrill (1998) has demonstrated how institutional entrepreneurs in the field of law were particularly successful at pressing for

change in the interstices of institutions to accomplish the acceptance of court-based alternative dispute resolution programs.

17. Joan Cassell (1998) makes a similar point in her book about the masculine culture of surgery.

CHAPTER 4

1. Meyerson 2003 [2001]; Meyerson and Scully 1995; Morrill, Zald, and Rao 2003; Scully and Segal 2002.

2. Dorothy Holland (1988) explains how expressions of emotion, language choice, and entry into particular spaces are claims to particular positions of privilege relative to others. When people claim positions to which they are seen to be unentitled, others are likely to rebuff their attempts.

3. It is interesting that I find little difference along racial lines in likelihood of being an internal reformer. The percentage of residents interviewed in my study—across all levels—who were internal reformers was 75 among White residents, 81 among Asian residents, and 83 among Black residents. We might have expected to see greater differences between white residents and minority residents, given the literature on race and medical education. This literature shows that 61 percent of racial minority medical students reported at least one experience of discrimination during US medical school in the form of racial slurs, being denied opportunities, and experiencing poor evaluations (Baldwin, Daugherty, and Rowly 1994). In addition, in surgical residency, racial minorities report being seen as not compulsive enough and not having the right cowboy mentality to get the job done; members of racial minorities are more likely to be terminated than white male residents, even when rank in the program is controlled for, and are less likely to be forgiven poor responses to criticism (O'Connell 2007). In contrast to O'Connell's race effect, in my sample the gender effect is considerably greater; the percentage of reformers among white men and minority men is essentially the same (69 percent of white men versus 71 percent of minority men). There is a slight race effect in the female sample, with 100 percent of the minority women at all levels (including interns) being reformers as compared to 89 percent of the white women. But even here, the differences by gender are considerably higher, with 100 percent reformers among minority women compared to 71 percent reformers among minority men.

4. Howard Becker and colleagues (1961, 1956a, and1956b) discuss how newcomers to the medical profession come in with other strongly held identifications, such as those growing out of participation in the family of orientation. Tensions arise when the new professional identity fails to mesh with or meet the specifications of these other identities. Over time, through interaction with others in the profession, new recruits develop pride in new skills, acquire professional ideology, and internalize motives. This results in attachment to occupational title, task commitment, and commitment to particular work organizations or positions in them.

5. Informants did have a term to describe these residents: "noncategorical

residents." Because this term is a bit unwieldy, I call them "other-specialty" residents instead. They included both residents in non–general surgical specialties such as urology, ENT, and ophthalmology and residents in specialties further afield such as emergency medicine and pathology.

6. Goffman 1961.

7. Readers may wonder whether there were biases in whom I chose to talk to and who chose to talk to me. The answer is no. At Advent and Bayshore, where I conducted ethnographic observation, I interviewed a very high percentage of residents (91 and 88 percent, respectively). At Calhoun, where I conducted ethnographic interviewing a year later, I interviewed a lower percentage (67 percent). There I targeted general surgery chiefs and interns for my interviews (and interviewed 100 percent of these), because I had learned that these residents were most important to the change effort; if they did not collaborate, I had found, change did not occur. In addition, I interviewed a selection of senior residents and other specialty interns. I spoke to senior residents who had been randomly assigned to the general surgery rotations during the time I was conducting the pre-interviews and to other specialty interns who had been randomly assigned to rotate first on the general surgery services.

8. Those who had several different reformer concerns tended to be especially strong supporters of reform.

9. Douglas Creed, Maureen Scully, and John Austin (2002) point out that internal reformers often need to tailor social movement frames for use in their own organizational settings.

10. Advent, Bayshore, and Calhoun had similar numbers of senior and chief resident reformers (10, 11, and 11 respectively) and similar numbers of interns who were beneficiaries of change (20, 23, and 20 respectively). To be conservative, these numbers do not include the chief and senior residents who were not interviewed prior to the change effort. If these residents were counted based on how I observed or others reported they acted in the free spaces of cafeterias and call rooms, the count would be 11 for Advent, 12 for Bayshore, and 15 for Calhoun.

CHAPTER 5

1. John Van Maanen details how newcomers to organizations experience and commit themselves to a new way of life replete with particular rules of thumb, standards of conduct, and customs and rituals suggestive of how members are to relate to colleagues and superiors (Van Maanen 1976; Van Maanen and Barley 1984).

2. June 2002 at Advent and Bayshore and June 2003 at Calhoun.

3. At the time, I found this threat of retribution by the director ironic since the directors supported change. However, the threat that a director would hear about it if an intern acted up was a well-worn trope of residency training, and it is likely that McLaughlin used it here out of habit or because he had given the same speech in previous years.

4. At Advent and Bayshore, where programs were introduced the year before

changes were officially mandated, the directors decided *not* to monitor the new program closely by requiring residents to use timesheets to report their weekly work hours. Had they done so, the ACGME could have demanded to see these timesheets during their site visits, and directors wanted to determine how best to implement the new system before tracking it in a way that the regulatory agency could follow. At Calhoun, where the program was introduced the year the changes were mandated, directors tracked resident work hours using the official timesheets required by the ACGME. But everyone knew that these official timesheets did not reflect reality. At Calhoun, as at hospitals across the country, residents reported the hours they knew the ACGME wanted to see rather than those they actually worked.

5. Kolb and Putnam 1992; Morrill 1989; Morrill 1995; Morrill, Zald, and Rao 2003.

CHAPTER 6

1. For more detail, see Kellogg 2009.
2. Fantasia and Hirsch 1995; Gamson 1996; Polletta 1999.
3. Gamson 1992b.
4. Patricia Ewick and Susan Silbey (2003) explain how stories of resistance enable collective challenge.
5. Gamson 1992a; Polletta and Jasper 2001; Taylor and Whittier 1992.
6. Snow and Benford 1988; Snow et al. 1986.
7. It is interesting that the reformers did not point out that the residents had also always shared work with nurses, lab employees, and therapists. Perhaps to preserve their own professional status, even reformers referred to the work done by these groups as less important to the care of patients.
8. Patients are more acute now because cost-containment measures have led to a reduced length of stay after surgery and the shifting of many formerly hospitalized patients to ambulatory surgery.
9. Joyce Fletcher (1999) discusses how crucial teamwork behaviors can become labeled "being nice." In her study, women did relational work to get the project done but were assumed to be doing it to be nice or because that's what women do. In fact, the women's behaviors were critical to accomplishing project goals, and this is what motivated them to act collaboratively, but their competence and contributions were not recognized and labeled as such.

CHAPTER 7

1. The concept of "countermobilization" implies intentionality on the part of the Iron Men. It is important, therefore, to consider how much Iron Man action was deliberate and self-conscious and recognized as a movement and how much of it was me, a sociologist, recognizing and identifying and naming patterns in their behavior. Most interpretation in interaction is implicit. It becomes explicit as an active, conscious matter only when novel

situations are experienced or when our assumptions about situational rules are challenged (e.g. Van Maanen 2001). Active interpretation of the actions of the self and others is a common phenomenon only when persons are showered with unexpected, sometimes traumatic experiences that violate their sense of routine, normality or propriety. I suggest that the reformers' attacks represented challenges to accepted situational rules and routines and so sparked Iron Man reflexivity and intentional judgment about the reformers' actions.

2. They did not tell stories of male residents doing so even though no residents were in the hospital twenty-four hours a day, seven days a week. Male residents who were not in the hospital were often assumed to be doing something work- related (such as practicing surgery at the surgical simulation lab or doing lab work related to academic papers), while female residents who were not in the hospital were assumed to be at home taking care of their partner or children.

3. Gamson 1990 [1975]; McCarthy and Zald 1977; Tilly 1978.

4. Brueggemann 2000; Kurtz 2002; McCammon and Campbell 2002; Meyer and Staggenborg 1996; Staggenborg 1986; Van Dyke and Cress 2006.

5. Readers may wonder whether divisive countertactics played a role in the quick defeat of reform at Bayshore, since Bayshore had both the highest percentage of female residents and a similar percentage of women in chief positions to that of Calhoun. It did not. Divisive countertactics were not necessary at Bayshore because reformers there never mounted an organized and sustained challenge to defenders.

CHAPTER 8

1. Institutional theorists have demonstrated that for new practices to become accepted, they must be legitimated or deemed appropriate by field actors within a socially constructed system of norms, values, and beliefs. Richard Scott (2007) has highlighted three different kinds of legitimacy—regulative, normative, and cognitive—and Mark Suchman (1995) has discussed how actors can construct legitimacy for a new practice. John Sutton and Frank Dobbin (1996) have shown that peripheral actors may initiate a new practice and more central actors may later legitimate it.

2. In fact, during the prior resident year, I had often observed interns checking on patients after this named three hour cutoff period. Patients were taken care of post-operatively by highly trained critical care nurses in the recovery room, and often interns were busy and not able to check in on them within three hours.

3. Eliot Freidson (1970, 1986) discusses how physicians do not criticize other physicians outside of their professional circle.

CONCLUSIONS AND IMPLICATIONS

1. IOM 2008.

2. Landrigan et al. 2006.

3. Of course the ACGME has national data on compliance aggregated from individual programs, but residents have been shown to underreport their work hours to the ACGME. See Britt et al. 2009; IOM 2008.

4. IOM 2008, 6.

5. Ibid.

6. ACS 2008.

7. AMSA 2008; CIR 2008; Public Citizen 2008.

8. Public Citizen 2008, 1.

9. AMSA 2008; Public Citizen 2008.

10. DiMaggio and Powell 1983; Scott 2007.

11. For example, Stephen Barley and colleagues, in ethnographic studies of radiology technicians, emergency medical technicians, and contractors, recount how frontline actors in organizations are critical to wielding ideas and lodging claims that alter institutions (Barley 1986; Barley 2008; Barley and Kunda 2004; Barley and Tolbert 1997; Nelsen and Barley 1997). For other studies of the importance of frontline actors to institutional change, see Dacin and Dacin 2008; Hallett and Ventresca 2006; Lawrence and Suddaby 2005; Munir and Phillips 2005; Orlikowski and Iacono 2000; Reay, Golden-Biddle, and Germann 2006.

12. For example, in their analysis of thirty-one years of technology transfer archives at Stanford University, Jeanette Colyvas and Walter Powell (2006, 2007, 2008) detail how individuals in concrete social situations change institutions by giving traditional practices new meanings and recombining already established routines to normalize new activities.

13. For example, Tammar Zilber (2002), in her ethnographic study of a rape crisis center, explains how the influx of new staff members with a therapeutic rather than feminist ideology was critical to accomplishing change in long-standing practices. See also Battilana and Dorado (forthcoming) for an analysis of the importance of new staff to institutional change.

14. For a review of this literature, see Edelman and Petterson 1999.

15. In their studies of what leads top managers to adopt new programs, law and society theorists do not make this mistake. For example, in their studies of the adoption of compliance programs, law and society theorists such as Frank Dobbin (2009) and Lauren Edelman (1990) note the importance of industry-level normative and cognitive understandings in shaping top manager decisions to adopt compliance programs.

16. Felstiner, Abel, and Sarat 1981.

17. Edelman, Erlanger, and Lande 1993; Harlan and Robert 1998; Marshall 2005.

18. For example, Erin Kelly and Alexandra Kalev (2006) have demonstrated that workers often do not even attempt to use flexible work arrangements established for their benefit by top managers unless their direct supervisors support their right to do so. For other studies of the importance of direct supervisor support for compliance program use, see Albiston 2005; Blair-Loy and Wharton 2002; Blair-Loy and Wharton 2004; Edelman, Erlanger, and Lande 1993; Edelman, Fuller, and Mara-Drita 2001; Fuller, Edelman, and Matusik 2000; Harlan and Robert 1998; Marshall 2005.

19. For reviews of the ways that external reformers can promote social change inside organizations, see Davis et al. 2005; Davis et al. 2008; McAdam and Scott 2005; Rao, Morrill, and Zald 2000; Zald, Morrill, and Rao 2005.

20. Mayer Zald, Calvin Morrill, and Hayagreeva Rao (2005) discuss the importance of top managers to implementing social movement reform inside organizations.

21. For studies demonstrating the importance of internal reformer access to external and internal resources to the implementation of social change inside organizations, see Creed and Scully 2000; Dutton and Ashford 1993; Lounsbury 2001; Meyerson 2003 [2001]; Meyerson and Scully 1995; O'Mahony and Bechky 2008; Scully and Segal 2002.

22. For example, Mary Katzenstein (1998) demonstrates how the different political opportunities available to women in the military versus women in the church have led the two groups of activists to fight in different ways for change inside their organizations: women in the military have used interest-group politics while women in the church have used discursive protests. For other accounts of how internal reformers accomplish change using classic social movement processes, see the foundational study by Mayer Zald and Michael Berger (1978) and more recent studies: Binder 2002; Briscoe and Safford 2008; Creed, Scully, and Austin 2002; Kaplan 2008; Kurtz 2002; Moore 2008; Raeburn 2004; Weber, Thomas, and Rao 2009.

23. For example, in her study of the mobilization of lesbian, gay, and bisexual employee networks to win domestic partner benefits in Fortune 1000 companies, Nicole Raeburn (2004) shows that the success of intra-organizational movements depends on the external and political and cultural opportunities available to activists inside organizations. In a different study of intra-organizational mobilization, Klaus Weber, LG Thomas, and Hayagreeva Rao (2009) demonstrate that the effect of the anti-genetic movement was conditioned by organizations' internal polities.

24. Healthcare social movements often challenge existing medical practice as they fight for expanded healthcare access or improved patient safety (e.g., Banaszak-Holl, Levitsky, and Zald 2010; Brown and Zavestoski 2005; Taylor 1996).

25. Abbott 1988; Freidson 1986; Starr 1982.

26. Abbott 1988; Larson 1977.

27. Stefan Timmermans and Marc Berg (2003) discuss how the movement toward evidence-based medicine can be seen as an attempt by physicians to regain the public's trust and safeguard the profession's position by emphasizing the scientific foundation of their work. They introduce the helpful distinction between "professional autonomy" (the profession's control over entrance to the field, self-monitoring, developing a body of specialized knowledge, and running professional organizations) and "clinical autonomy" (the individual practitioner's control over routine work activities and decisions) to explain this phenomenon. They suggest that we should not be surprised by the discrepancy between increasing rhetoric around evidence-based medicine on the one hand and limited actual change in clinical practice on the other; by introducing new standards and then not

enforcing these standards in practice, physicians maintain both collective control over their professional jurisdiction and individual control over their daily work.

28. For instance, in their study of neo-natal units, Carol Heimer and Lisa Staffen demonstrate that hospital providers and state agents implement medical regulation differently in everyday interactions because of their different interests and their different definitions of infants' problems and potential solutions (Heimer 1999; Heimer and Staffen 1998).

29. For example, Robert Zussman (1992) shows how ICU physicians protect their professional authority in the face of informed-consent mandates by turning moral questions into questions of technical expertise. Similarly, Renee Anspach (1993) explains how NICU physicians guard their autonomy by preempting parental resistance, persuading parents to adopt their point of view, and neutralizing parental dissent.

30. Heimer 1999; Timmermans and Berg 2003.

31. Medical sociologists have not neglected the importance of organizational factors to reform implementation altogether. For example, Daniel Chambliss (1996) demonstrates that nurses' failure to even recognize when they are making ethnical decisions arises from their subordinate position to physicians in the hospital bureaucracy. Similarly, Renee Anspach (1993) and Charles Bosk (1992) note that nurses and genetic counselors, respectively, play more minor roles in bioethics decision making than do NICU physicians because nurses' and counselors' subordinate positioning in the organizational hierarchy results in their knowledge claims being discounted. However, these theorists have not explained how variation in organizational resources shapes variation in reform outcomes across organizations.

32. Conrad 2008.

33. IOM 2008.

34. Ibid.

35. Mary Bernstein (1997) has made a similar point about the celebration and suppression of identity.

36. In order to prevent a splintering of the internal reformer collective, external reformers would also need to promote practices that build solidarity— for example, by developing language and demeanor that are common to reformers across subgroups. Sharon Kurtz (2002) talks about this idea of building common practices across diverse social identity groups.

37. Alexandra Kalev, Erin Kelly, and Frank Dobbin (2006) make a similar point in their study of civil rights law implementation about the importance of assigning accountability for change.

38. IOM 2008, 229–30.

39. Ibid., 231.

40. Ibid., 232.

41. Frank Dobbin and Alexandra Kalev (2007) and Emilio Castilla and Stephen Benard (2009) similarly suggest that appearing to favor groups who have been traditionally discriminated against can lead to backlash.

42. Meyerson 2003 [2001].

References

Abbott, A. 1988. *The system of professions: An essay on the division of expert labor.* Chicago: University of Chicago Press.

ACGME (Accreditation Council for Graduate Medical Education). 2004. The ACGME's approach to limit resident duty hours 12 months after implementation: A summary of achievements. Vol. 2004. Available at http://www.acgme.org/acWebsite/dutyHours/dh_dutyhoursummary2003-04.pdf.

ACS (American College of Surgeons). 2008. American College of Surgeons comments on Institute of Medicine report on resident duty hours. Press release, December 3. http://www.facs.org/education/statement.pdf.

Albiston, C. 2005. Bargaining in the shadow of social institutions: Competing discourses and social change in workplace mobilization of civil rights. *Law and Society Review* 39 (1): 11–49.

Alexander, V. 1996. Pictures at an exhibition: Conflicting pressures in museums and the display of art. *American Journal of Sociology* 101 (4): 797–839.

AMSA (American Medical Student Association). 2008. "Medical students react to IOM Report: Resident work hours reexamined." Press release, December 2. Available at http://www.amsa.org/AMSA/Homepage/About/News/News11.aspx.

Anderson, C., R. Albrecht, K. Anderson, and R. Dean. 1996. Can continuity-of-care requirements for surgery residents be demonstrated in the current teaching environment? *Archives of Surgery* 131 (9): 915–21.

Andrews, A. 1995. I was juror no. 6, the lone dissenter in the Libby Zion case. *New York Times*, February 21.

Anspach, R. 1993. *Deciding who lives: Fateful choices in the intensive care nursery.* Berkeley: University of California Press.

Anteby, M. 2008. Identity incentives as an engaging form of control: Revisiting leniencies in an aeronautic plant. *Organization Science* 19 (2): 202–20.

Association of American Medical Colleges. 2009. AAMC survey of resident/fellow stipends and benefits. Autumn.

Bailyn, L. 2006 [1993]. *Breaking the mold: Redesigning work for productive and satisfying lives.* 2nd ed. New York: Cornell University Press.

Baker, T. 2007. *The medical malpractice myth.* Chicago: University of Chicago Press.

Baldwin, D., S. Daugherty, and B. Rowly. 1994. Emotional impact of medical school and residency: Racial and ethnic discrimination during residency; Results of a national survey. *Academic Medicine* 69 (10).

Banaszak-Holl, J., S. Levitsky, and M. Zald. 2010. *Social movements and the transformation of American health care.* New York: Oxford University Press.

Barley, S. 1986. Technology as an occasion for structuring: Evidence from observations of CT scanners and the social order of radiology departments. *Administrative Science Quarterly* 31 (1): 78–108.

———. 1996. Technicians in the workplace: Ethnographic evidence for bringing work into Organization Studies. *Administrative Science Quarterly* 41 (3): 404–41.

———. 2008. Coalface institutionalism. In R. Greenwood, C. Oliver, R. Suddaby, and K. Sahlin-Andersson (eds.), *The SAGE handbook of organizational institutionalism.* Thousand Oaks, CA: Sage.

Barley, S. R., and G. Kunda. 2004. *Gurus, hired guns, and warm bodies: Itenerant experts in a knowledge economy.* Princeton, NJ: Princeton University Press.

Barley, S. R., and P. S. Tolbert. 1997. Institutionalization and structuration: Studying the links between action and institution. *Organization Studies* 18 (1): 93–117.

Barnard, A. 2002. Surgery residents' long hours draw warning for Yale. *Boston Globe*, May 20, Metro/Region sec., 1.

Baron, J., F. Dobbin, and P. Jennings. 1986. War and peace: The evolution of modern personnel administration in United States industry. *American Journal of Sociology* 92 (2): 350–83.

Battilana, J., and S. Dorado. Forthcoming. Building sustainable hybrid organizations: The case of commercial microfinance organizations. *Academy of Management Journal.*

Becker, H. 1960. Notes on the concept of commitment. *American Journal of Sociology* 66:32–40.

———. 1961. *Boys in white: Student culture in medical school.* Chicago: University of Chicago Press.

Becker, H., and J. Carper. 1956a. The development of identification with an occupation. *American Journal of Sociology,* 61 (4): 289–98.

———. 1956b. The elements of identification with an occupation. *American Journal of Sociology* 21:341–48.

Bell, B. 2003. Reconsideration of the New York State laws rationalizing the supervision and the working conditions of residents. *Einstein Journal of Biology and Medicine* 20:36–40.

Bernstein, M. 1997. Celebration and suppression: The strategic uses of identity by the lesbian and gay movement. *American Journal of Sociology* 103 (3): 531–65.

Binder, A. 2002. *Contentious curricula: Afrocentrism and creationism in American public schools.* Princeton, NJ: Princeton University Press.

Bird, C., P. Conrad, A. Fremont, and S. Timmermans. 2010. *Handbook of medical sociology.* 6th ed. Nashville: Vanderbilt University Press.

Blackbourne, L. 1996. *Advanced surgical recall.* Baltimore: Williams and Wilkins.

Blair-Loy, M., and A. Wharton. 2002. Employees' use of work-family policies and the workplace social context. *Social Forces* 80 (3): 813–45.

———. 2004. Organizational commitment and constraints on work-family policy use: Corporate flexibility policies in a global firm. *Sociological Perspectives* 47 (3): 243–67.

Boodman, S. G. 2001. Sleep deprived residents, interns admit to lax care. *Los Angeles Times,* April 16.

Bosk, C. 1992. *All God's mistakes: Genetic counseling in a pediatric hospital.* Chicago: University of Chicago Press.

———. 2003 [1979]. *Forgive and remember: Managing medical failure.* 2nd ed. Chicago: University of Chicago Press.

Briscoe, F., and S. Safford. 2008. The Nixon-in-China effect: Activism, imitation, and the institutionalization of contentious practices. *Administrative Science Quarterly* 53 (3): 460–91.

Britt, L., A. Sachdeva, G. Healy, T. Whalen, and P. Blair. 2009. Resident duty hours in surgery for ensuring patient safety, providing optimum resident education and training, and promoting resident well-being: A response from the American College of Surgeons to the report of the Institute of Medicine, "Resident duty hours: enhancing sleep, supervision, and safety." *Surgery* 146:398–409.

Brosnan, C., and B. Turner. 2009. *Handbook of the sociology of medical education.* London: Routledge.

Brown, P., and S. Zavestoski, eds. 2005. *Social movements in health.* Malden, MA: Blackwell.

Brueggemann, J. 2000. The power and collapse of paternalism: The Ford Motor Company and black workers, 1937–1941. *Social Problems* 47 (2): 220–40.

Bucher, R., and J. Stelling. 1977. *Becoming professional.* Beverly Hills, CA: Sage.

Carper, J., and H. Becker. 1957. Adjustments to conflicting expectations in the development of identification with an occupation. *Social Forces* 36:212–23.

Cassell, J. 1998. *The woman in the surgeon's body.* Cambridge, MA: Harvard University Press.

Castilla, E., and S. Benard. 2009. The paradox of meritocracy: Hidden risks in merit-based performance systems. Paper presented at the annual meeting of the American Sociological Association, San Francisco, August 8.

Chambliss, D. 1996. *Beyond caring: Hospitals, nurses, and the social organization of ethics.* Chicago: University of Chicago Press.

Chang, A. 2004. Group says new doctors work fewer hours. Associated Press Online, July, 28.

CIR (Committee of Interns and Residents). 2008. CIR welcomes the Institute of Medicine's report which calls for 16-hour maximum shifts for patient care. Press release, December 2.

Clemens, E. 1993. Organizational repertoires and institutional change: Women's groups and the transformation of United States politics, 1890–1920. *American Journal of Sociology* 98 (4): 755–98.

———. 2005. Two kinds of stuff: The current encounter of social movements and organizations. In G. F. Davis, D. McAdam, W. R. Scott, and M. N. Zald (eds.), *Social movements and organization theory*, 351–66. Cambridge: Cambridge University Press.

Clemens, E., and J. Cook. 1999. Politics and institutionalism: Explaining durability and change. *Annual Review of Sociology* 25 (1): 441–66.

Colburn, D. 1988. Medical education: Time for reform? After a patient's death, the 36-hour shift gets new scrutiny. *Washington Post*, March 29.

Colyvas, J. 2007. From divergent meanings to common practices: The early institutionalization of technology transfer in the life sciences at Stanford University. *Research Policy* 36 (4): 456–76.

Colyvas, J., and W. W. Powell. 2006. Roads to institutionalization: The remaking of boundaries between public and private science. In *Research in organizational behavior: An annual series of analytical essays and critical reviews*, vol. 27, ed. B. Staw, 305–53. Greenwich, CT: JAI Press.

Conrad, P. 1988. Learning to doctor: Reflections on recent accounts of the medical school years. *Journal of Health and Social Behavior* 29 (4): 323–32.

———. 2008. *The sociology of health and illness*. 8th ed. New York: Worth.

Conrad, P., and J. Schneider. 1992. *Deviance and medicalization: From badness to sickness*. St. Louis: Temple University Press.

Creed, W., and M. Scully. 2000. Songs of ourselves: Employees' deployment of social identity in workplace encounters. *Journal of Management Inquiry* 9 (4): 391–412.

Creed, W., M. Scully, and J. Austin. 2002. Clothes make the person? The tailoring of legitimating accounts and the social construction of identity. *Organization Science* 13 (5): 475–96.

Czeisler, C. 2009. It's time to reform work hours for resident physicians. *Science-News* 176 (9): 36.

Dacin, M. T., and P. A. Dacin. 2008. Traditions as institutionalized practice: Implications for de-institutionalization. In R. Greenwood, C. Oliver, R. Suddaby, and K. Sahlin-Andersson (eds.), *The SAGE Handbook of Organizational Institutionalism*. Thousand Oaks, CA: Sage.

D'Aunno, T., M. Succi, and J. Alexander. 2000. The role of institutional and market forces in divergent organizational change. *Administrative Science Quarterly* 45 (4): 679–703.

Davis, G., and H. Greve. 1997. Corporate elite networks and governance changes in the 1980s. *American Journal of Sociology* 103 (1): 1–37.

Davis, G., D. McAdam, W. Scott, and M. Zald, eds. 2005. *Social movements and organization theory*. Cambridge: Cambridge University Press.

Davis, G., C. Morrill, H. Rao, and S. Soule. 2008. Introduction: Social movements in organizations and markets. *Administrative Science Quarterly* 53 (3): 389–94.

DiMaggio, P. J. 1988. Interest and agency in institutional theory. In L. G. Zucker (ed.), *Institutional patterns and organizations: Culture and environment*, 3–21. Cambridge, MA: Ballinger.

———. 1991a. Constructing organizational field as a professional project: U.S. art museums, 1920–1940. In W. W. Powell and P. DiMaggio (eds.), *The new institutionalism in organizational analysis*, 267–92. Chicago: University of Chicago Press.

———. 1991b. Expanding the scope of institutional analysis. In W. W. Powell and P. J. DiMaggio (eds.), *The new institutionalism in organizational analysis*, 190–203. Chicago: University of Chicago Press.

DiMaggio, P. J., and W. W. Powell. 1983. The iron cage revisited: Institutional isomorphism and collective rationality in organizational fields. *American Sociological Review* 48 (2): 147–60.

Dobbin, F. 2009. *Inventing equal opportunity*. Princeton, NJ: Princeton University Press.

Dobbin, F., L. Edelman, J. Meyer, W. Scott, and A. Swidler. 1988. The expansion of due process in organizations. In L. Zucker (ed.), *Institutional patterns and organizations: Culture and environment*, 71–100. Cambridge, MA: Ballinger.

Dobbin, F., and A. Kalev. 2007. The architecture of inclusion: Evidence from corporate diversity programs. *Harvard Journal of Law and Gender* 30 (2): 279–301.

Dobbin, F., and E. Kelly. 2007. How to stop harassment: Professional construction of legal compliance in organizations. *American Journal of Sociology* 112 (4): 1203–43.

Dobbin, F., J. Sutton, J. Meyer, and W. Scott. 1993. Equal opportunity law and the construction of internal labor markets. *American Journal of Sociology* 99: 396–427.

Douglas, R. 1995. Zion case verdict vindicates training system. *New York Times*, February 14.

Drummond, S., et al. 2000. Altered brain response to verbal learning following sleep deprivation. *Nature* 403 (6770): 655–57.

Dunn, M., and R. Miller. 1997. US graduate medical education, 1996–1997. *JAMA* 278 (9): 750–54.

Dutton, J., and S. Ashford. 1993. Selling issues to top management. *Academy of Management Review* 18 (3): 397–428.

Edelman, L. 1990. Legal environments and organizational governance: The expansion of due process in the American workplace. *American Journal of Sociology* 95 (6): 1401–40.

———. 1992. Legal ambiguity and symbolic structures: Organizational mediation of civil-rights law. *American Journal of Sociology* 97 (6): 1531–76.

Edelman, L., S. Abraham, and H. Erlanger. 1992. Professional construction of the legal environment: The inflated threat of wrongful discharge doctrine. *Law and Society Review* 26 (1): 47–83.

Edelman, L., H. Erlanger, and J. Lande. 1993. Internal dispute resolution: The transformation of civil rights in the workplace. *Law and Society Review* 27 (3): 497–534.

Edelman, L., S. Fuller, and I. Mara-Drita. 2001. Diversity rhetoric and the managerialization of law. *American Journal of Sociology* 106 (6): 1589–641.

Edelman, L., and S. Petterson. 1999. Symbols and substance in organizational response to civil rights law. *Research in Social Stratification and Mobility* 17: 107–35.

Edelman, L., S. Petterson, E. Chambliss, and H. Erlanger. 1991. Legal ambiguity and the politics of compliance: Affirmative action officers' dilemma. *Law and Policy* 13 (1): 73–97.

Edelman, L., and R. Stryker. 2005. A sociological perspective on law and the economy. In N. Smelser and R. Swedberg (eds.), *Handbook of economic sociology*, 2nd ed., 527–51. Princeton, NJ: Princeton University Press.

Edelman, L., and M. Suchman. 1997. The legal environments of organizations. *Annual Review of Sociology* 23:479–515.

Edelman, L., C. Uggen, and H. Erlanger, 1999. The endogeneity of legal regulation: Grievance procedures as rational myth. *American Journal of Sociology* 105 (2): 406–54.

Ewick, P., and S. Silbey. 2003. Narrating social structure: Stories of resistance to legal authority. *American Journal of Sociology* 108 (6): 1328–72.

Fantasia, R., and E. Hirsch. 1995. Culture in rebellion: The appropriation and transformation of the veil in the Algerian revolution. In H. Johnston and B. Klandermans (eds.), *Social movements and culture*, 4:144–59. Minneapolis: University of Minnesota Press.

Felstiner, W., R. Abel, and A. Sarat. 1981. The emergence and transformation of disputes: Naming, blaming, claiming. *Law and Society Review* 15 (3–4): 631–54.

Fine, G. 1996. Justifying work: Occupational rhetorics as resources in restaurant kitchens. *Administrative Science Quarterly* 41 (1): 90.

Fletcher, J. 1999. *Disappearing acts: Gender, power, and relational practice at work.* Cambridge, MA: MIT Press.

Fligstein, N. 1985. The spread of the multidivisional form among large firms, 1919–1979. *American Sociological Review* 50 (3): 377–91.

———. 1997. Social skill and institutional theory. *American Behavioral Scientist* 40 (4): 397–405.

Fox, R. 1957. Training for uncertainty. In R. K. Merton, G. Reader, and P. Kendall (eds.), *The student-physician: Introductory studies in the sociology of medical education*, 207–41. Cambridge, MA: Harvard University Press.

———. 1959. *Experiment perilous: Physicians and patients facing the unknown.* Glencoe, IL: Free Press.

Fox-Wolfgramm, S., K. Boal, and J. Hunt. 1998. Organizational adaptation to institutional change: A comparative study of first-order change in prospector and defender banks. *Administrative Science Quarterly* 43 (1): 87–126.

Freidson, E. 1970. *Professional dominance: The social structure of medical care.* New York: Atherton.

———. 1986. *Professional powers: A study of institutionalization of formal knowledge.* Chicago: University of Chicago Press.

———. 1988. *Profession of medicine: A study of the sociology of applied knowledge.* Chicago: University of Chicago Press.

Friedland, R., and R. Alford. 1991. Bringing society back in: Symbols, practices, and institutional contradictions. In W. W. Powell and P. J. DiMaggio (eds.), *The new institutionalism in organizational analysis*, 232–63. Chicago: University of Chicago Press.

Friedman, R., J. Bigger, and D. Kornfield. 1971. The intern and sleep loss. *New England Journal of Medicine* 285:201–3.

Fuller, S., L. Edelman, and S. Matusik. 2000. Legal readings: Employee interpretation and mobilization of law. *Academy of Management Review* 25 (1):
200–216.

Gaba, D., and S. Howard. 2002. Fatigue among clinicians and the safety of patients.
New England Journal of Medicine 347 (16): 1249–55.

Galison, P., and D. Stump. 1996. *The disunity of science: Boundaries, contexts, and
power.* Stanford, CA: Stanford University Press.

Gamson, W. 1988. Political discourse and collective action. *International Social
Movement Research* 1:219–44.

———. 1990 [1975]. *The strategy of social protest.* Belmont, CA: Wadsworth.

———. 1992a. The social psychology of collective action. In A. Morris and C. Mueller (eds.), *Frontiers in social movement theory,* 53–76. New Haven, CT: Yale
University Press.

———. 1992b. *Talking politics.* New York: Cambridge University Press.

———. 1996. Safe spaces and social movements. *Perspectives on Social Problems*
8:27–38.

Garrett, S. 1995. An effective dose of scrutiny. *Washington Post,* September 12.

Glaser, B., and A. Strauss. 1967. *The discovery of grounded theory: Strategies for qualitative research.* Chicago: Aldine.

Goffman, E. 1956. The nature of deference and demeanor. *American Anthropologist*
58 (3): 475–99.

———. 1961. *Asylums: Essays on the social situation of mental patients and other in-
mates.* Garden City, NY: Anchor Books.

Grantcharov, T., L. Bardram, P. Funch-Jensen, and J. Rosenberg. 2001. Laparoscopic
performance after one night on call in a surgical department: Prospective
study. *BMJ* 323:1222–23.

Greening, D., and B. Gray. 1994. Testing a model of organizational response to social and political issues. *Academy of Management Journal* 37 (3): 467–98.

Greenwood, R., C. Oliver, R. Suddaby, and K. Sahlin-Andersson, eds. 2008. *The
SAGE handbook of organizational institutionalism.* Thousand Oaks, CA: Sage.

Greenwood, R., and R. Suddaby. 2006. Institutional entrepreneurship in mature
fields: The big five accounting firms. *Academy of Management Journal* 49 (1):
27–48.

Greenwood, R., R. Suddaby, and C. Hinings. 2002. Theorizing change: The role
of professional associations in the transformation of institutionalized fields.
Academy of Management Journal 45 (1): 58–80.

Grunebaum, A., H. Minkoff, and D. Blake. 1987. Pregnancy among obstetricians: A
comparison of births before, during, and after residency. *American Journal of
Obstetrics and Gynecology* 157:79–83.

Guillén, M. 1994. *Models of management: Work, authority, and organization in a comparative perspective.* Chicago: University of Chicago Press.

Hafferty, F., and D. Light. 1995. Professional dynamics and the changing nature of
medical work. *Journal of Health and Social Behavior* 35:132–53.

Hallett, T., and M. Ventresca. 2006. Inhabited institutions: Social interactions and
organizational forms in Gouldner's *Patterns of Industrial Bureaucracy. Theory and Society* 35 (2): 213–36.

Hardy, C., and S. Maguire. 2008. Institutional entrepreneurship. In R. Greenwood, C. Oliver, R. Suddaby, and K. Sahlin-Andersson (eds.), *The SAGE Handbook of Organizational Institutionalism*, 198–217. Thousand Oaks, CA: Sage.

Harlan, S., and P. Robert. 1998. The social construction of disability in organizations: Why employers resist reasonable accommodation. *Work and Occupations* 25 (4): 397–435.

Harris Interactive. 2009. Harris survey on occupational prestige. Available at http://www.harrisinteractive.com/vault/Harris-Interactive-Poll-Research-Pres-Occupations-2009-08.pdf.

Harrison, Y., and J. Horne. 2000. The impact of sleep deprivation on decision making: A review. *Journal of Experimental Psychology: Applied* 6 (3): 236–49.

Haveman, H., and H. Rao. 1997. Structuring a theory of moral sentiments: Institutional and organizational coevolution in the early thrift industry. *American Journal of Sociology* 102 (6): 1606–51.

Haveman, H., Rao, H., & Paruchuri, S. 2007. The winds of change: The progressive movement and the bureaucratization of thrift. *American Sociological Review* 72 (1): 117–42.

Heimer, C. 1996. Explaining variation in the impact of law: Organizations, institutions, and professions. *Studies in Law, Politics and Society* 15:29–59.

———. 1999. Competing institutions: Law, medicine, and family in neonatal intensive care. *Law and Society Review* 33 (1): 17–66.

Heimer, C., and L. Staffen. 1998. *For the sake of the children: The social organization of responsibility in the hospital and the home.* Chicago: University of Chicago Press.

Hinings, C., R. Greenwood, T. Reay, and R. Suddaby. 2004. Dynamics of change in organizational fields. In M. Poole and A. Van de Ven (eds.), *Handbook of organizational change and innovation*, 304–23. London: Oxord University Press.

Holland, D., W. Lachicotee, D. Skinner, and C. Cain. 1988. *Identity and agency in cultural worlds.* Cambridge, MA: Harvard University Press.

Hughes, E. 1971. *The sociological eye.* Chicago: Aldine-Atherton.

Hunt, S., R. Benford, and D. Snow. 1994. Identity fields: Framing processes and the social construction of movement identities. In L. Johnston, and J. Gusfield (eds.), *New social movements: From ideology to identity.* Philadelphia: Temple University Press.

IOM (Institute of Medicine). 2008. Resident duty hours: Enhancing sleep, supervision, and safety. Washington, DC: National Academies Press.

Jasper, J. M., and F. Polletta. 2001. Collective identity and social movements. *Annual Review of Sociology* 27:283–305.

Kalev, A., and F. Dobbin. 2006. Enforcement of civil rights law in private workplaces: The effects of compliance reviews and lawsuits over time. *Law and Social Inquiry: Journal of the American Bar Foundation* 31 (4): 855–903.

Kalev, A., F. Dobbin, and E. Kelly. 2006. Best practices or best guesses? Assessing the efficacy of corporate affirmative action and diversity policies. *American Sociological Review* 71:589–617.

Kalev, A., Y. Shenhav, and D. De Vries. 2008. The state, the labor process, and the diffusion of managerial models. *Administrative Science Quarterly* 53 (1): 1–28.

Kaplan, S. 2008. Framing contests: Strategy making under uncertainty. *Organization Science* 19 (5): 729–52.

Katz, P. 1999. *The scalpel's edge: The culture of surgeons.* Boston: Allyn and Bacon.

Katzenstein, M. 1998. *Faithful and fearless: Moving feminist protest inside the church and military.* Princeton, NJ: Princeton University Press.

Kellogg, K. 2009. Operating room: Relational spaces and microinstitutional change in surgery. *American Journal of Sociology* 115 (3): 657–711.

Kelly, E. 2003. The strange history of employer-sponsored child care: Interested actors, uncertainty, and the transformation of law in organizational fields. *American Journal of Sociology* 109 (3): 606–49.

———. 2010. Failure to update: An institutional perspective on noncompliance with the family and medical leave act. *Law and Society Review* 44 (1): 33–66.

Kelly, E., and F. Dobbin. 1998. How affirmative action became diversity management: Employer response to antidiscrimination law, 1961 to 1996. *American Behavioral Scientist* 41 (7): 960–84.

———. 1999. Civil rights law at work: Sex discrimination and the rise of maternity leave policies. *American Journal of Sociology* 105 (2): 455–92.

Kelly, E., and A. Kalev. 2006. Managing flexible work arrangements in US organizations: Formalized discretion or "a right to ask." *Socio-economic Review* 4 (3): 379.

Kennedy, R. 1998. Residents' hours termed excessive in hospital study. *New York Times*, May 19.

King, B. 2008. A political mediation model of corporate response to social movement activism. *Administrative Science Quarterly* 53 (3): 395–421.

King, B., and S. Soule. 2007. Social movements as extra-institutional entrepreneurs: The effect of protests on stock price returns. *Administrative Science Quarterly* 52 (3): 413–42.

Klebanoff, M., P. Shiono, and G. Rhoads. 1990. Outcomes of preganancy in a national sample of resident physicians. *New England Journal of Medicine* 323:1040–45.

Kleitman, N. 1963. *Sleep and wakefulness.* Chicago: University of Chicago Press.

Kolb, D., and L. Putnam, eds. 1992. *Hidden conflict in organizations: Uncovering behind-the-scenes disputes.* Thousand Oaks, CA: Sage.

Kowalenko, T., J. Haas-Kowalenko, A. Rabinovich, and M. Grzybowski. 2000. Emergency medicine residency related MVCs—is sleep deprivation a risk factor? *Academic Emergency Medicine* 7 (5): 451.

Kurtz, S. 2002. *Workplace justice: Organizing multi-identity movements.* Minneapolis: University of Minnesota Press.

Laine, C., L. Goldman, J. Soukup, and J. Hayes. 1993. The impact of regulation restricting medical house staff working hours on the quality of patient care. *JAMA* 269:374–78.

Landrigan, C., L. Barger, B. Cade, N. Ayas, and C. Czeisler. 2006. Interns' compliance with accreditation council for graduate medical education work-hour limits. *JAMA* 296 (9): 1063–70.

Landrigan, C., J. Rothschild, J. Cronin, R. Kaushal, E. Burdick, J. Katz, C. Lilly, P. Stone, S. Lockley, D. Bates, and C. Czeisler. 2004. Effect of reducing interns' work hours on serious medical errors in intensive care units. *New England Journal of Medicine* 351 (18): 1838–48.

Larson, M. 1977. *The rise of professionalism: A sociological analysis.* Berkeley: University of California Press.

Lawrence, T., and R. Suddaby. 2005. Institutions and institutional work. In S. Clegg, C. Hardy, T. Lawrence, and W. Nord (eds.), *Handbook of organization studies*, 2nd ed. London: Sage.

Light, D. 1980. *Becoming psychiatrists: The professional transformation of self.* New York: W. W. Norton .

———. 2000. The medical profession and organizational change: From professional dominance to countervailing power. In C. Bird, P. Conrad, and A. Fremont (eds.), *Handbook of Medical Sociology*, 201–16. Upper Saddle River, NJ: Prentice Hall.

Lounsbury, M. 2001. Institutional sources of practice variation: Staffing college and university recycling programs. *Administrative Science Quarterly* 46 (1): 29–56.

Lounsbury, M., M. Ventresca, and P. Hirsch. 2003. Social movements, field frames and industry emergence: A cultural-political perspective of U.S. recycling. *Socio-economic Review* 1:71–104.

Marcus, C., and G. Loughlin. 1996. Effects of sleep deprivation on driving safety in housestaff. *Sleep* 19 (10): 763–66.

Marshall, A. 2005. Idle rights: Employees' rights consciousness and the construction of sexual harassment policies. *Law and Society Review* 39 (1): 83–123.

McAdam, D. 1999 [1982]. *Political process and the development of Black insurgency, 1930–1970.* Chicago: University of Chicago Press.

McAdam, D., J. McCarthy, and M. Zal. 1996. *Comparative perspectives on social movements: Political opportunities, mobilizing structures, and cultural framings.* Cambridge: Cambridge University Press.

McAdam, D., and W. Scott. 2005. Organizations and movements. In G. Davis, D. McAdam, W. Scott, and M. Zald (eds.), *Social movements and organization theory*, 4–40. Cambridge: Cambridge University Press.

McCall, T. 1988. The impact of long working hours on resident physicians. *New England Journal of Medicine* 318 (12): 775–78.

McCammon, H., and K. Campbell. 2002. Allies on the road to victory: Coalition formation between the suffragists and the Woman's Christian Temperance Union. *Mobilization* 7:231–51.

McCann, M. W. 1994. *Rights at work: Pay equity reform and the politics of legal mobilization.* Chicago: University of Chicago Press.

McCarthy, J., and M. Zald. 1977. Resource mobilization and social movements: A partial theory. *American Journal of Sociology* 82 (6): 1212–41.

McKinlay, J., and L. Marceau. 2002. The end of the golden age of doctoring. *International Journal of Health Services* 32 (2): 379–416.

Medical Group Management Association. 2009. Physician compensation and production survey. Available at http://www5.mgma.com/ecom/Default.aspx?tabid=138&action=INVProductDetails&args=4610.

Merton, R., G. Reader, and P. Kendall. 1957. *The student-physician: Introductory stud-*

ies in the sociology of medical education. Cambridge, MA: Harvard University Press.

Meyer, D., and S. Staggenborg. 1996. Movements, countermovements, and the structure of political opportunity. *American Journal of Sociology* 101 (6): 1628–60.

Meyer, J., and B. Rowan. 1977. Institutionalized organizations: Formal structure as myth and ceremony. *American Journal of Sociology* 83 (2): 340–63.

Meyerson, D. 2003 [2001]. *Tempered radicals: How everyday leaders inspire change at work.* Boston: Harvard Business School Press.

Meyerson, D., and M. Scully. 1995. Tempered radicalism and the politics of ambivalence and change. *Organization Science* 6:585–600.

Mezias, S. J. 1990. An institutional model of organizational practice: Financial-reporting at the Fortune 500. *Administrative Science Quarterly* 35 (3): 431–57.

Mezias, S. J., and M. Scarselletta. 1994. Resolving financial reporting problems: An institutional analysis of the process. *Administrative Science Quarterly* 39 (4): 654–78.

Mizrahi, T. 1986. *Getting rid of patients.* New Brunswick, NJ: Rutgers University Press.

Moore, K. 1996. Organizing integrity: American science and the creation of public interest organizations, 1955–1975. *American Journal of Sociology* 101 (6): 1592–627.

———. 2008. *Disrupting science: Social movements, American scientists, and the politics of the military.* Princeton, NJ: Princeton University Press.

Morrill, C. 1989. The management of managers: Disputing in an executive hierarchy. *Sociological Forum* 4 (3): 387–407.

———. 1995. *The executive way.* Chicago: University of Chicago Press.

———. 1998. The growth of alternative dispute resolution in American public and private sectors, 1965-1995." Paper presented at the Law & Society Association annual meeting, Snowmass, CO, June 4–7.

Morrill, C., M. Zald, and H. Rao. 2003. Covert political conflict in organizations: Challenges from below. *Annual Review of Sociology* 29:391–415.

Mukherjee, S. 2002. Resident aliens: Are medical residents working too hard? *New Republic* 227:14–18.

———. 2004. Becoming a physician: A precarious exchange. *New England Journal of Medicine* 351 (18): 1822–24.

Munir, K., and N. Phillips. 2005. The birth of the "Kodak moment": Institutional entrepreneurship and the adoption of new technologies. *Organization Studies* 26 (11): 1665–87.

Nelsen, B. J., and S. R. Barley. 1997. For love or money? Commodification and the construction of an occupational mandate. *Administrative Science Quarterly* 42 (4): 619–53.

Neumayer, L., et al. 2002. The state of general surgery residency in the United States: Program director perspectives, 2001. *Archives of Surgery* 137 (11): 1262–65.

New York State Department of Health. 1989. New York State Residency Working Hours and Hospital Code Regulations, 405.4 (b) (6). Albany, NY.

New York Supreme Court. 1986. Report of the Fourth Grand Jury for the April/May term of 1986 concerning the care and treatment of a patient and the supervision of interns and junior residents at a hospital in New York County. New York: Supreme Court of the State of New York, County of New York.

New York Times. 2002. Sleep-deprived doctors. June 14.

———. 2008. Napping during hospital shifts. December 9.

O'Connell, V. 2007. *Getting cut: Failing to survive surgical residency training.* New York: University Press of America.

O'Mahony, S., and B. Bechky. 2008. Boundary organizations: Enabling collaboration among unexpected allies. *Administrative Science Quarterly* 53 (3): 422–59.

Oliver, C. 1991. Strategic responses to institutional processes. *Academy of Management Review* 16 (1): 145–79.

———. 1992. The antecedents of deinstitutionalization. *Organization Studies*, 13 (4): 563–88.

Orlikowski, W., and S. Iacono, eds. 2000. *The truth is not out there: An enacted view of the "digital economy."* Cambridge, MA: MIT Press.

Palmer, D., P. Jennings, and X. Zhou. 1993. Late adoption of the multidivisional form by large United States corporations: Institutional, political, and economic accounts. *Administrative Science Quarterly* 38 (1): 100–131.

Parks, D., et al. 2000. Day-night pattern in accidental exposures to blood-borne pathogens among medical students and residents. *Chronobiology International* 17 (1): 61–70.

Patrick, G., and J. Gilbert. 1896. On the effects of loss of sleep. *Psychological Review* 3 (5): 469–83.

Perez-Pena, R. 1994. Nine years of resolve: Trial to begin in daughter's death. *New York Times*, November 1.

Petersen, L., et al. 1994. Does housestaff discontinuity of care increase the risk for preventable adverse events? *Annals of Internal Medicine* 121 (11): 866–72.

Phillips, D., and E. Zuckerman. 2001. Middle-status conformity: Theoretical restatement and empirical demonstration in two markets. *American Journal of Sociology* 107 (2): 379–429.

Pilcher, J., and A. Huffcutt. 1996. Effects of sleep deprivation on performance: A meta-analysis. *Sleep* 19:318–26.

Pitts, F., A. Schuller, C., Rich, and A. Pitts. 1979. Suicide among U.S. women physicians, 1967–1972. *American Journal of Pscyhiatry* 136:694–96.

Polletta, F. 1999. "Free spaces" in collective action. *Theory and Society* 28 (1): 1–38.

Polletta, F., and J. Jasper. 2001. Collective identity and social movements. *Annual Review of Sociology* 27:283–305.

Portas, C., et al. 1998. A specific role for the thalmus in mediating the interaction of attention and arousal in humans. *Journal of Neuroscience* 18 (21): 8979–89.

Powell, W. W. 1991. Expanding the scope of institutional analysis. In W. W. Powell and P. J. DiMaggio (eds.), *The new institutionalism in organizational analysis*, 183–203. Chicago: University of Chicago Press.

Powell, W. W., and J. Colyvas. 2008. Microfoundations of institutional theory. In R. Greenwood, C. Oliver, R. Suddaby, and K. Sahlin-Andersson (eds.), *The SAGE Handbook of Organizational Institutionalism*, 276–98. Thousand Oaks, CA: Sage.

Public Citizen. 2001. Petition to the Occupational Safety and Health Adminis-
    tration requesting that limits be placed on hours worked by medical resi-
    dents. Washington, DC: HRG Publication, April 30. Available at http://www
    .citizen.org/hrg1570.
————. 2008. Institute of Medicine Report on Resident Work Hours misses oppor-
    tunity, fails to endorse significant federal oversight. Washington, DC: HRG
    Publication. December 2. Available at http://www.citizen.org/pressroom/
    pressroomredirect.cfm?ID=2777.
Quadagno, J. 2004. Why the United States has no national health insurance: Stake-
    holder mobilization against the welfare state, 1945–1996. *Journal of Health
    and Social Behavior* 45:25–44.
Raeburn, N. 2004. *Inside out: The struggle for lesbian, gay, and bisexual rights in the
    workplace.* Minneapolis: University of Minnesota Press.
Rao, H., P. Monin, and R. Durand. 2003. Institutional change in Toque Ville: Nou-
    velle cuisine as an identity movement in French gastronomy. *American Jour-
    nal of Sociology* 108 (4): 795–843.
————. 2005. Border crossing: Bricolage and the erosion of categorical boundaries
    in French gastronomy. *American Sociological Review* 70 (6): 968–91.
Rao, H., C. Morrill, and M. Zald. 2000. Power plays: How social movements and
    collective action create new organizational forms. In B. Staw and R. Sutton
    (eds.), *Research in organizational behavior,* vol. 22, 237–81. New York: JAI–
    Elsevier Science.
Reay, T., K. Golden-Biddle, and K. Germann. 2006. Legitimizing a new role: Small
    wins and microprocesses of change. *Academy of Management Journal* 49 (5):
    977–98.
Reuben, D. 1985. Depressive symptoms in medical house officers: Effects of level of
    training and work rotation. *Archives of Internal Medicine* 145:286–88.
Ridgeway, C. Forthcoming. *Framed by gender: How gender inequality persists in the
    modern world.* New York: Oxford University Press.
Rosoff, S., and M. Leone. 1991. The public prestige of medical specialties: Over-
    views and undercurrents. *Social Science and Medicine* 32 (3): 321–26.
Rubinowitz, S. 1999. You're sick and they're tired: Hospital horror stories from ex-
    hausted docs. *New York Post.*
Samkoff, J., and C. Jacques. 1991. A review of studies concerning effects of sleep
    deprivation and fatigue on residents' performance. *Academic Medicine* 66:
    687–93.
Scott, W. 2007. *Institutions and organizations: Ideas and interests.* 3rd ed. Thousand
    Oaks, CA: Sage.
Scott, W., M. Ruef, P. Mendel, and C. Caronna. 2000. *Institutional change and
    healthcare organizations: From professional dominance to managed care.* Chi-
    cago: University of Chicago Press.
Scully, M. A., and A. Segal. 2002. Passion with an umbrella: Grassroots activists
    in the workplace. In M. Lounsbury and M. J. Ventresca (ds.), *Research in the
    sociology of organizations,* 127–70. Oxford: JAI Press.
Seo, M., and W. Creed. 2002. Institutional contradictions, praxis, and institutional
    change: A dialectical perspective. *Academy of Management Review* 27 (2):
    222–47.

Silbey, S. 1981. Case processing: Consumer protection in an attorney general's office. *Law and Society Review* 15 (3–4): 849–81.

Silbey, S., R. Huising, and S. Coslovsky. 2009. The sociological citizen: Recognizing relational interdependence in law and organizations. *Année Sociologique* 59 (1): 201–29.

Snow, D., and R. Benford. 1988. Ideology, frame resonance, and participant mobilization. *International Social Movement Research* 1:197–217.

Snow, D., E. Rochford, S. Worden, and R. Benford. 1986. Frame alignment processes, micromobilization, and movement participation. *American Sociological Review* 51:464–81.

Soule, S. 2009. *Contention and corporate responsibility*. Cambridge: Cambridge University Press.

Spradley, J. 1979. *The ethnographic interview*. New York: Holt Rinehart and Winston.

Staggenborg, S. 1986. Coalition work in the pro-choice movement: Organizational and environmental opportunities and obstacles. *Social Problems* 33 (5): 375–90.

Starr, P. 1982. *The social transformation of American medicine*. New York: Basic Books.

Steele, M., et al. 1999. The occupational risk of motor vehicle collisions for emergency medicine residents. *Academic Emergency Medicine* 610:1050–53.

Steinbrook, R. 2002. The debate over residents' work hours. *New England Journal of Medicine* 347 (16): 1296–302.

Strang, D., and D. I. Jung. 2005. Organizational change as an orchestrated social movement: Recruitment to a corporate quality initiative. In G. F. Davis, D. McAdam, W. R. Scott, and M. N. Zald (eds.), *Social movements and organization theory*. Cambridge: Cambridge University Press.

Strazouso, J. 2004. Young doctors working too many hours. Associated Press.

Suchman, M. 1995. Managing legitimacy: Strategic and institutional approaches. *Academy of Management Review* 20 (3): 571–611.

Suchman, M., and L. Edelman. 2007. The interplay of law and organizations. In L. Edelman and M. Suchman (eds.), *The legal lives of private organizations*, 1–49. Aldershot, UK: Ashgate.

Sutton, J., and F. Dobbin. 1996. The two faces of governance: Responses to legal uncertainty in U.S. firms, 1955 to 1985. *American Sociological Review* 61 (October): 794–811.

Sutton, J., F. Dobbin, J. Meyer, and W. Scott. 1994. The legalization of the workplace. *American Journal of Sociology* 99 (4): 944–71.

Swidler, A. 2001. *Talk of love: How culture matters*. Chicago: University of Chicago Press.

Tarrow, S. 1994. *Power in movement: Social movements, collective action, and politics*. Cambridge: Cambridge University Press.

Taylor, M., and M. Zald. 2010. Conclusion: The shape of collective action in the U.S. health sector. In J. Banaszak-Holl, S. Levitsky, and M. Zald (eds.), *Social movements and the transformation of American health care*. New York: Oxford University Press.

Taylor, V. 1996. *Rock-a-by baby: Feminism, self-help, and postpartum depression.* New York: Routledge.

Taylor, V., and N. Raeburn. 1995. Identity politics as high-risk activism: Career consequences for lesbian, gay, and bisexual sociologists. *Social Problems* 42 (2): 252–73.

Taylor, V., and N. Whittier. 1992. Collective identity in social movement communities: Lesbian feminist mobilization. In A. Morris and C. Mueller (eds.), *Frontiers in social movement theory,* 104–30. New Haven, CT: Yale University Press.

Thomas, M., et al. 2000. Neural basis of alertness and cognitive performance impairments during sleepiness: Part 1, Effects of 24 h of sleep deprivation on waking human regional brain activity. *Journal of Sleep Research* 9 (4): 335–52.

Tilly, C. 1978. *From mobilization to revolution.* Reading, MA: Addison-Wesley.

Timmermans, S., and M. Berg. 2003. *The gold standard: The challenge of evidence-based medicine and standardization in health care.* Philadelphia: Temple University Press.

Tolbert, P. S., and L. G. Zucker. 1983. Institutional sources of change in the formal structure of organizations: The diffusion of civil service reform, 1880–1935. *Administrative Science Quarterly* 28 (1): 22–39.

———. 1996. The institutionalization of institutional theory. In S. Clegg, C. Hardy, and W. R. Nord (eds.), *Handbook of organization studies,* 175–90. Thousand Oaks, CA: Sage.

US Bureau of Labor Statistics. 2002. Occupational employment statistics. Washington, DC: Government Printing Office.

US Congress. 2001. Patient and Physician Safety and Protection Act of 2001—Amends Title XVIII (Medicare) of the Social Security Act (SSA) to require a participating hospital that uses the services of physician residents or postgraduate trainees to limit their working hours to specified schedules, 107th Congress, 1st Session. Washington, DC.

US Congressional Research Service. 2007. U.S. health care spending: Comparison with other OECD countries. Washington, DC: Government Printing Office.

Valko, R., and P. Clayton. 1975. Depression in internship. *Diseases of the Nervous System* 36:26–29.

Van Dyke, N., and R. Cress. 2006. Political opportunities and collective identity in Ohio's gay and lesbian movement, 1970 to 2000. *Sociological Perspectives* 49 (4): 503–26.

Van Maanen, J. 1976. Breaking in: Socialization to work. In R. Dubin (ed.), *Handbook of work, organization, and society,* 67–101. Chicago: Rand McNally College.

———. 1988. *Tales of the field: On writing ethnography.* Chicago: University of Chicago Press.

———. 2001. *Identity work: Notes on the personal identity of police officers.* Paper presented at the annual meeting of the Academy of Management, San Diego, CA, August 9–1.

Van Maanen, J., and S. Barley. 1984. Occupational communities: Culture and control in organizations. *Research in Organizational Behavior* 6:287–365.

Vaughan, D. 1996. *The Challenger launch decision: Risky technology, culture, and deviance at NASA*. Chicago: University of Chicago Press.

Veasey, S., et al. 2002. Sleep loss and fatigue in residency training: A reappraisal. *JAMA* 288:1116–24.

Weber, K., L. Thomas, and H. Rao. 2009. From streets to suites: How the anti-biotech movement affected German pharmaceutical firms. *American Sociological Review* 74 (1): 106–27.

Weinger, M., and S. Ancoli-Israel. 2002. Sleep deprivation and clinical performance. *JAMA* 287:955–57.

Westphal, J., and E. Zajac. 1994. Substance and symbolism in CEOs' long-term incentive plans. *Administrative Science Quarterly* 39 (3): 367–90.

Whang, E., M. Mello, S. Ashley, and M. Zinner. 2003. Implementing resident work hour limitations: Lessons from the New York State experience. *Annals of Surgery* 237 (4): 449–55.

Whyte, W. 1949. The social structure of the restaurant. *American Journal of Sociology* 54 (4): 302–10.

Zald, M. 2008. Epilogue: Social movements and political sociology in the analysis of organizations and markets. *Administrative Science Quarterly* 53 (3): 568–74.

Zald, M., and M. Berger. 1978. Social movements in organizations: Coup d'etat, insurgency, and mass movements. *American Journal of Sociology* 83 (4): 823–61.

Zald, M., C. Morrill, and H. Rao. 2005. The impact of social movements on organizations: Environment and responses. In G. Davis, D. McAdam, W. Scott, and M. Zald (eds.), *Social movements and organization theory*, 253–79. New York: Cambridge University Press.

Zeigler, J. 2004. Caught squealing: Physician whistleblowers voice concerns about hospital care, often to find themselves targeted instead. *New Physician* 53 (9).

———. 2005. We've only just begun: Two hours after work-hours regulations implementation, programs—and residents—slowly adjust. *New Physician* 54 (4).

Zetka, J. 2003. *Surgeons and the scope*. Ithaca, NY: Cornell University Press.

Zilber, T. 2002. Institutionalization as an interplay between actions, meanings, and actors: The case of a rape crisis center in Israel. *Academy of Management Journal* 45 (1): 234–54.

Zinner, M. 2002. Surgical residencies: Are we still getting the best and the brightest? Pamphlet. Boston: Brigham and Women's Hospital.

Zussman, R. 1992. *Intensive care: Medical ethics and the medical profession*. Chicago: University of Chicago Press.

Index

Abbott, Andrew, 12, 198n9

ABSITE (American Board of Surgery In-Training Examination). *See* American Board of Surgery In-Training Examination (ABSITE)

accreditation, threatened loss of, 33–34

ACGME (American Council for Graduate Medical Education). *See* American Council for Graduate Medical Education (ACGME)

administrators. *See* directors

Advanced Surgical Recall (textbook), 56

Advent Hospital (pseud.): afternoon rounds at, 117, 121–22, 129; challenge of status quo at, 8; characteristics of, 39–40; coalition building at, 172; collective disruption at, 148–53, 169; countermovement threat at, 139–40; cross-position challenges at, 126–27; defenders' capitulation at, 147–48, 158; desire for work-life balance at, 37; divisive countertactics at, 136–38; facilitating defender accommodation at, 153–57; lack of subgroup threat at, 140–41, 144, 168–69, 173; legitimating new practices at, 158–61; outrage of defenders at, 135–36; persistence of reformers at, 144; reformers' coalition at, 17; relational mobilization at, 123–26, 130–31; reputation of residency program

at, 134; research methods and, 7–8, 14–16, 194n80, 200n7, 200n10; success of reformer coalition at, 138–40

Alexander, Jeffrey, 198–99n16

Alford, Robert, 198–99n16

AMA (American Medical Association). *See* American Medical Association (AMA)

American Board of Surgery In-Training Examination (ABSITE), 162

American College of Surgeons, 3–4, 166

American Council for Graduate Medical Education (ACGME): accreditation and, 5, 43; action against noncompliant hospitals by, 165; announcement of work-hours regulations by, 33, 167; attending physicians' anger at, 42; compliance monitoring and, 166, 180–81, 200–201n4; enforcement power of, 167; external pressure on, 43; jurisdiction over reform and, 5; professional self-regulation and, 178, 180; underreporting of hours to, 165, 203n3; whistleblower protections and, 180–81; work-hours guidelines of, 5–7

American Medical Association (AMA), 12

American Medical Student Association (AMSA), 3, 43, 166, 180–81

AMSA. *See* American Medical Student Association (AMSA)